Psycholo... D0446793

HERE TO HELP

secrets of
SUCCESSFUL
WEIGHT LOSS

Diana Burrell

ALPHA

A member of Penguin Group (USA) Inc.

For Oliver.

Contents

Foreword

Just walk down the street, and you will find that the statistics are spot-on. More than 64 percent of American adults are overweight or dangerously obese. That's a staggering number. In fact, issues of weight are just as acute among our young—some 15 percent of children are overweight. And it's a problem that isn't going away. But the good news is issues regarding diet and weight start at the top—in your mind.

Granted, your mind can be your worst enemy—when faulty thinking and negative self-talk push you toward junk food and mega-portions. Beyond that, one's mood can also wreak havoc on the waistline. We all know the story: we turn to food to cope with life's stresses; we eat when we're depressed; we eat when our relationships turn sour. And we override our best intentions when we are just plain mentally exhausted. It's no surprise most of us have an unhealthy relationship with food.

Yet *Secrets of Successful Weight Loss* shows you that your mind can be your greatest ally. In fact, your mind is *the* key to your success. This book gives you the tools you need to identify the triggers and feelings that drive you to unhealthy eating habits. It's a reinvention of sorts, where you learn how to approach your diet and weight differently. And for some of us, losing the weight is one thing, but keeping it off is another. It is not about forfeiting all the foods you love for 2 months and then going back to "normal" eating.

Sure there are quick fixes, fad diets, lifestyle approaches, and clinically supervised plans. But how do all these methods work, and what diet is right for you? This book deconstructs the vast variety of options available for you to make the choice that best suits you. It also shows you the importance of living right—through exercise, getting a good night's rest, and finding the support you need.

Author Diana Burrell gives us a comprehensive guide in these pages. As an experienced journalist, she is well qualified to write this book. Not only has she covered this topic a great deal, but she has had her own battles with weight as well. From her first-hand knowledge, she shows us that this is not just a weight-loss book; it's a handbook that will help you rethink your relationship with food, weight, and diet. This is the book that will give you the insight you need to live a healthier, happier life.

Kaja Perina
Editor in chief
Psychology Today

Introduction

Let me first admit that for most of my life, I've been thin. Thin, but not healthy. While many of my friends were on every diet imaginable to lose their excess pounds, my metabolism coped with whatever I threw at it. And most of what I threw at it wasn't very healthful: a lot of candy, coffee, and junk food, the occasional vegetable (I disliked animal protein), and a minimal amount of exercise. No wonder by the time I turned 30 I was battling chronic exhaustion as well as a budding weight problem.

I visited several doctors who tried to figure out what was wrong with me. Only one doctor asked about my diet, and when I admitted I subsisted largely on sugar and caffeine, she ordered a glucose-tolerance test. Halfway through the 3-hour blood test, I fainted in the waiting room. Diagnosing me as severely hypoglycemic, she put me on a diet of frequent meals of high-fat, high-protein foods.

For someone like me who didn't have a clue about healthy eating, this diet prescription spelled disaster for my weight. It was carte blanche to eat scrambled eggs dripping in butter, dump cream over my fruit, and snack on as much cheese as I liked. During the low-fat craze of the 1990s, my "diet" made me a pariah among my friends. It also made me a lot fatter.

I knew overweight was becoming a problem when I asked my doctors not to tell me what the scale said during routine physicals. Or I'd get photos developed and hide the "fat pictures" before my husband could see them. I stopped wearing shorts in the summer and started all kinds of diets. I did Atkins. I joined a gym and followed the Body for Life plan. I dropped in on a couple Weight Watchers meetings. I tried detox diets and food combining, and even took ephedra after a fellow writer told me how she'd lost 30 pounds on it. Whatever diet I tried would work for a couple weeks. I'd lose 5 or 10 pounds. But then I'd get bored or hungry or just tired of drinking my breakfast, lunch, and dinner, and I'd go right back to my careless eating habits—and gain more weight.

My (new) family physician did me a huge favor when he pulled out a weight chart and showed me that I'd officially joined the 64 percent of Americans who are overweight. I was nearing 40 and feeling it, especially because I was exhausted chasing an active toddler around the house. On top of that, my total blood cholesterol was high. I was tired of feeling fat, tired of feeling unfit, tired of feeling tired. Not only did I want to lose weight, but I wanted to be healthy, too. And I didn't want to have to go on some "diet" for the rest of my life to achieve these two goals.

In less than a year, I lost all the weight I'd gained in the past 10 years—more than 35 pounds. My history of yo-yo dieting had showed me how my mind worked, if there was any good news to be found there. I knew a diet labeling certain foods "bad" wouldn't fly with me—my brain is especially resistant to denial. Any plan that required a gym membership got nixed: I loathe every minute I'm indoors on a stair-stepper. And if I were to join a support group, it would have to be online because of my family and work schedules.

My love of cooking and experimenting with new tastes let me expand my repertoire of healthful meals. Portion control is something I can live with as long as I don't have to deal with denial. And I love to walk—not only does it give my heart a good workout, but walking makes me feel better physically *and* emotionally.

The answer for me—and I believe for anyone who wants to lose weight healthily and permanently—was to minimize the roadblocks my mind put up during a diet and to capitalize on its immense power. What it comes down to for most successful dieters is less about what goes into their mouths—the actual diet—and more about what goes on between their ears—what they bring to that diet. Successful weight loss is understanding how you respond to such triggers as stress, hunger, emotions, and holidays—and following a plan that gets you through these moments. It's figuring out an eating and exercise plan that fits into the life you have today, not the one you think you'll have tomorrow. It's learning how to focus on long-term benefits versus short-term gratification. Successful weight loss is all about mastering the awesome power of your brain.

And we're here to help you.

Whether you've got 10 or 15 stubborn pounds around your midsection or you've battled serious overweight and obesity your whole life, *Secrets of Successful Weight Loss* guides you through the tangled emotions, urges, thoughts, and feelings that can make dieting so difficult. You learn what research says about certain diets and get a feel for which eating and exercise plan will work best for you. After you've created your weight-loss plan, I give you the best tips, tricks, and tools others have used to stay moti-vated and stick the course. You learn how to deal with setbacks and why it's important to celebrate victories. And I share with you some of the benefits, as well as challenges, you can look for-ward to with permanent weight loss. Best of all, you meet inspir-ing men and women of all ages and backgrounds who've been able to lose weight and keep it off.

What You'll Find Inside This book is organized in four parts:

In **Part 1: "Mind Over Matter,"** you discover how the mind is your secret ally—as well as its unwitting saboteur—when you're trying to lose weight. You learn why you're attracted to quick fixes, and what psychological traits successful dieters tend to share.

In **Part 2, "Weight Loss That Works for You,"** I give you an overview of all the different types of diets out there today, from plans based on restriction and lifestyle, to fad diets and plans supervised by doctors and clinicians.

In **Part 3, "Working the Plan,"** you learn how to design a diet and exercise plan that works for you—everything from choosing the foods you eat to how you monitor yourself—as well as what to do about plateaus, setbacks, and rewards. You also learn about some secret weapons that successful dieters have used to remain motivated.

In the last section, **Part 4, "Beyond the Diet,"** I show you how successful weight loss improves your health. You also discover how to ask for help—and how to offer help to other dieters as well. And because I'm confident you'll lose the weight you set out to lose, I share with you some of the mental adjustments you'll want to make with permanent weight loss.

How to Use This Book This book was written to be read from beginning to end. But if you're anything like me, you're a grazer. So go ahead—flip to the last chapter. Reading about what it's like to lose weight and keep it off might inspire you to turn back to the beginning and to learn how your mind responds to change—especially when it comes in the form of food.

If you're already dieting and dealing with some psychological challenges, this book is set up so you can quickly turn to the sections that have the most relevance for you. For example, if you're having a tough time coping with lack of support during the holiday season, there's a chapter about finding support (Chapter 14) and separate sections about handling sabotage and holidays.

Nearly every page of this book includes boxes or notes that highlight important advice, inspiration, and personal stories that add to the chapter. Don't skip them! As I wrote them, I imagined you picking up this book and looking for something to keep you focused on your plan. Think of these bonus boxes as healthy snacks for your mind:

In Q&A sidebars, you get expert answers to important questions about weight loss.

PsychSpeak

PsychSpeak sidebars spell out difficult or unfamiliar terms in plain English. A glossary at the back of the book contains even more definitions.

GET PSYCHED

Get Psyched notes include important motivational nuggets you need to remember, all from successful dieters and weight-loss experts.

WEB TALK sidebars point you to helpful websites where you can get more information about the topic at hand.

you're not alone

You're Not Alone sidebars tell the inspiring story of a man or woman—someone like you—who has lost weight and kept it off.

Welcome to *Secrets of Successful Weight Loss* I am confident that when you understand how to get your brain to work with you on a diet, you'll end up spending less time "dieting" and more time enjoying life. Every successful dieter I interviewed for this book admitted they're much happier today than they were when they were overweight or obese. It's not because they're now "thin" and can fit into a size 4, although for some people, that's certainly a boon. But it's how weight loss makes them feel *inside:* confident, happy, and proud of their hard work and achievements. It's a feeling I want you to feel, too.

Acknowledgments First, a big thanks to *Psychology Today*'s Lybi Ma and Hara Estroff Marano, whose enthusiasm sold me on this project and made my participation possible. Huge thanks to everyone at Alpha Books who worked on this book—including Paul Dinas, Christy Wagner, Billy Fields, Tricia Liebig, Rebecca Harmon, and Donna Martin.

There are so many people in my life to thank. There's Melanie Glunz, who took such great care of my son so I could focus on work. Mark Davidson, M.D., who took such good care of *me* while I was writing this book. The Byline Babes—you girls kept me sane. Other friends and family deserve thanks for their support: Gwen Moran, Kate Stiffle, Sarah Smith, Linda Formichelli, Jane Gardner, Alison Stein Wellner, Matt Burrell, and Peter Schurman. My mother, Agnes, and my stepmother, Jan, who cheerfully babysat my son when I needed time to work. My father, John, who dropped his lab glassware to answer my late-night biochemistry questions. A special thanks to my mother-in-law, Elise Lawton, R.D., Ph.D., a woman whose intelligence and resourcefulness never cease to amaze me.

My son, Oliver, is my biggest inspiration. His optimism makes me believe all things are possible. I thank him for all the times he understood "it's Mommy's time to work." And this book would not be possible were it not for my husband, a Mac genius as well as a great sounding board.

I'm especially grateful to the experts I spoke with for this book, some of whom gave me hours of their time on evenings and weekends to answer my questions:

Edward Abramson, Ph.D., professor of psychology, California State University, Chico and author

Tammy Colter, director of operations at ObesityHelp.com

Lisa Dorfman, R.D., American Dietetic Association spokesperson and Miami-based sports nutritionist, licensed psychotherapist, and author

Mark Davidson, M.D.

Darwin Deen, M.D., professor of clinical family and social medicine at the Albert Einstein College of Medicine, Bronx, New York, and author

John W. Erdman Jr., Ph.D., professor of nutrition, department of food science and human nutrition, University of Illinois at Urbana-Champaign

Osama Hamdy, M.D., director of the Obesity Clinic and assistant investigator in the section on clinical research at Joslin Diabetes Center, an instructor in medicine at Harvard Medical School, Boston, and author

Susan Jeffers, Ph.D.

Victoria Moran

Robert Kushner, M.D., medical director of the Wellness Institute at Northwestern Memorial Hospital, Chicago, and author

Russell A. LaForte, M.D., director of the Center for Weight Management at University of Texas Medical Branch/Galveston

Elena M. Ramirez, Ph.D., clinical assistant professor of psychology at the University of Vermont in Burlington and a licensed psychologist-doctorate

Caroline Rudnick, M.D., Ph.D., St. Louis University School of Medicine

Most of all, I am grateful to and humbled by the amazing men and women who shared their stories of weight loss with me. These people overcame everything from unyielding genetics and bad habits to yo-yo dieting and morbid obesity. Their stories touched me deeply and motivated me on my own weight-loss journey. Many, many thanks.

Part 1

Mind Over Matter

When we diet, we tend to focus more on the food—the matter—
and less on what matters—the mind. In these initial chapters,
you learn why your brain is the most important tool you have
for successful weight loss.

The Missing Link in Weight-Loss Success

When you think about going on a diet, the first question you ask yourself is probably something such as *What do I have to eat to lose weight?* The next questions are usually along the lines of *How much can I eat? What* can't *I eat?* and *How long do I have to stay on this diet before I see results?* Many of us even think *And when can I go back to eating normal food?*

As you talk to diet experts or read weight-loss books, you might wonder if an improper mix of proteins, carbohydrates, and fats has led to your weight problem. Perhaps you should cut carbs because you adore bread and pasta. Or maybe you wonder if you even *want* to lose weight—after all, diets are misery.

What most people don't think about as they're contemplating diet and weight loss is the role of their own thoughts, feelings, beliefs, and attitudes in the success or failure of a weight-loss plan. They think more about what the diet brings to them and less about what they bring to the diet.

Think about it. Last time you went on a diet, did you pay more attention to weighing your food or weighing your thoughts? How much time did you spend forcing yourself to fit into a one-size-fits-all diet versus making the diet mesh with your personality and preferences?

Perhaps it's one reason why we see escalating numbers of Americans growing heavier each year. We certainly aren't at a loss for solid weight-loss programs; many of them do work and work well when they're followed. Rather, we seem to credit our success or failure with a diet to the *diet*, when we should be looking to *ourselves* for the diet's success or failure.

Your Mind: The Key to Successful Weight Loss

The statistics about overweight and obesity in America are daunting. According to the National Center for Health Statistics (NCHS) of the Centers for Disease Control and Prevention (CDC) in Maryland:

64 percent of adults age 20 and over are either overweight or obese with a body mass index (BMI) greater than 25. A full 30 percent of adults age 20 and over are obese, meaning they have a BMI greater than 30. BMI is a formula and equals a person's weight in kilograms divided by height in meters squared (BMI=kg/m^2).

Overweight and obesity are becoming more prevalent among both genders, smokers as well as nonsmokers, and across racial, ethnic, and educational levels. Whereas many public health problems all but disappeared in the twentieth century, overweight and obesity continue to claim more lives.

Our nation's children are very vulnerable to being overweight and obese. Approximately 15.3 percent of children ages 6 to 11 and 15.5 percent of adolescents ages 12 to 19 are overweight. An additional 15 percent of children and 14.9 percent of adolescents were at risk for overweight, with a BMI for their age between the 85th and 95th percentiles.

Q&A

What's the difference between overweight and obesity?

According to the Centers for Disease Control (CDC), someone who is overweight has a BMI of 25 to 29.9. Someone who is obese has a BMI of 30 to 39.9. A person whose BMI is greater than or equal to 40 is considered morbidly obese. A healthy BMI is between 20 and 25. A person who has increased muscle mass may qualify as overweight based on their BMI. However, the CDC points out that this is not overfat, which is the key factor in developing some serious health conditions. BMI calculation is only one tool in determining overweight or obesity. Other considerations include body fat measurement, waist-to-hip ratio, and waist measurement.

Most Americans are aware of the cost of overweight and obesity to their health and would like to do something about it. According to the American Obesity Association, a Washington, D.C.–based nonprofit organization, approximately 40 percent of women and 25 percent of men are attempting to lose weight at any given time. They estimate we spend $30 billion each year on products and programs that will help us attain the sometimes-elusive goal of losing weight and getting in shape. We spend money buying diet books that tell us which foods help us burn fat faster. We spend hours making sure our diet's ratio of carbs to fats and proteins is correct. Yet few of us spend much time or thought on the role our mind has in losing weight and how we can harness its power, no matter what eating plan we choose.

Why Do *You* Want to Lose Weight?

Your doctor may be urging you to lose some weight, your spouse might be encouraging you to stop snacking, and your kids could be begging you to run around the yard or play with them more after school. However, these may not be compelling enough reasons for you to embark on yet another diet plan. You may go through the motions and lose a few pounds, but you might do it just to please these people. If you're losing weight for someone else, you're not doing it for *you*. You really have to develop a strong and meaningful imperative that motivates you to take action—*for you*.

I interviewed dozens of successful "losers" for this book and asked them all why they finally decided to lose their weight. Their responses were often immediate, and although a great number of them had kept their weight off for years, their reasons for losing the weight were still fresh and often expressed with a great deal of emotion.

Their reasons are as unique as fingerprints:

One mother of two young children said she didn't want her children to grow up with an obese mother. She wanted them to have a mother who was fit, active, and fun—unlike the mother she had growing up.

A single, 20-something male said being obese became too tiring for him. He constantly worried about his appearance, his hygiene, and how others perceived him. After a humiliating incident at work, he was spurred to investigate surgical options for weight loss.

A woman on the verge of retirement said she was depressed and tired of feeling ashamed of her body. She wanted to wear cute clothes and play more golf with her friends.

Other dieters were told by their doctors they had to lose weight because of other health problems. They were, in effect, given a choice between life or death, and these people chose life.

A 40-ish executive mentioned she wanted to wear sexy, low-slung jeans and look better than her 20-year-old self in them. (She reports she does.)

It didn't seem to matter how serious or how silly the interviewees' reasons for finally losing their weight were. What mattered was that for these people, their reasons were strong enough to either get them started on a weight-loss program or continue on one, even if they started out less than motivated.

Dieters often start weight-loss programs without really knowing why they're doing so. They say, "I'm too heavy," or "I should lose weight." Well, those whys aren't very compelling, and such lackluster enthusiasm will rarely carry anyone very far on a diet. If you're vague about the reasons you want to lose weight, grab a piece of paper or open up a file in your word processor and answer the following questions. Be as specific as you can, and be honest with yourself in your answers:

- What pain do you associate with losing weight? For example, you may associate losing weight with being ravenously hungry all the time, missing out on your favorite foods, or having to stay home while your friends party on the weekends.

- What pleasure have you gained by not losing weight? Some examples: you get to eat all the food you want, you don't have to think about portion control, or you don't have to make time for exercise.

- What will the cost be if you don't start losing weight? For example, you may worry your spouse will find you less attractive as you grow heavier, or that you'll develop more serious health problems that could shorten your life.

- What will you gain if you do lose weight? Make this list long and exciting. How will you feel? What activities will you do? What kind of clothes will you wear? How will you enjoy life when you're fitter and healthier?

What are the health risks of overweight or obesity?

People who are overweight or obese are more likely to develop the following:

- Hypertension (high blood pressure)
- High total cholesterol
- High levels of triglycerides
- Type 2 diabetes
- Coronary heart disease
- Stroke
- Gallbladder disease
- Osteoarthritis
- Sleep apnea and respiratory problems
- Some cancers, such as endometrial, breast, and colon

If you're overweight or obese, weight loss can help reduce your chances of developing these health conditions. Studies show that a mere 5 to 10 percent reduction in weight can improve health.

(From the Centers for Disease Control and Prevention website on overweight and obesity, www.cdc.gov/nccdphp/dnpa/obesity/index.htm, April 24, 2005)

After this exercise, you should have a better idea of why you want to lose weight. If you don't feel very enthusiastic about your whys, come back to this exercise in a few days. Letting the questions simmer can often bring about an epiphany. For example, you might pick up the paper one morning and read an article about prejudice with overweight and obese workers. This may trigger a realization that you may have been passed over for a promotion because of your weight. This realization could be your "why": you no longer want to have your good work ignored.

A caution to this exercise: it's a good idea to pick a "why" that will benefit you over the long term. There's nothing wrong with wanting to lose weight to fit into your gown on your wedding day. But what happens when the wedding day is over? Will you still be motivated to continue your weight maintenance? Perhaps a more effective why would be adding "… and remain healthy and fit so I can be a good example to our future children."

Barriers to Weight Loss

There's no one reason why people get overweight or obese. It would be nice to blame our genes, but research suggests that genes don't act on their own; they react with other influences to promote weight gain. You can't place fault with someone's socioeconomic status: overweight and obesity are problems for the rich as well as the poor. You can't point to aging or the fact you're a woman, because, look around—plenty of people older than you are slim and many women remain fit. And you can't credit behavior. People do not become overweight or obese because they lack willpower or self-control.

It would be nice if your doctor could say, "The reason why you have this weight problem is because of X," and hand you a prescription to fix it. Although your doctor can help you identify some of the factors leading to your weight gain, solving your problem is going to be up to you. You have to look at everything that plays a part in your overweight and obesity and then develop a plan that takes each factor into account.

Genetics Maybe your mother and grandmother struggled with their weight. You might have the same "beer belly" your father and his father had. If overweight and obesity are written in your genes, how much control over your weight do you really have?

If one or both of your parents are obese, you have a 25 to 30 percent chance of being obese yourself. That leaves a 70 to 75 percent chance you *won't* be obese. Genetics certainly influence how much you weigh; genes control how your body burns calories for energy and how your body stores fat.

As of late 2004, researchers studying the human obesity gene map at the Human Genomics Laboratory in Baton Rouge, LA, and other research institutions have associated or linked more than 600 genes, markers, and chromosomal regions with human obesity phenotypes. This means researchers may be able to isolate a gene that triggers weight gain and treat it with a therapy that blocks *expression* of the gene. Hundreds of genes are now associated with overweight and obesity, so coming up with therapies could take some time.

You also inherit your family's attitudes about food. This makes it more difficult to pinpoint how much of a role genetics play in your weight versus how much inherited

GET PSYCHED

"Genes are not destiny. Obesity can be prevented or can be managed in many cases with a combination of diet, physical activity, and medication."
—*The Office of Genomics and Disease Prevention, Centers for Disease Control, May 5, 2005*

PsychSpeak

Expression, in genetic terms, is the manifestation or detectable effect of a gene. When gene expression occurs, coded information within the gene is converted into the structures present and operating in a cell.

attitudes and environment play. For example, what if you had heavy parents who drilled it into your head that you should always clean your plate? Or if you had parents who rewarded you with food when you were good or took it away when you were bad? What if you learned from your mother that the only way to lose weight (and not very effectively) was through crash dieting? Or what if your family was mostly sedentary, preferring to sit around the television at night rather than doing something physical together such as taking a walk?

Even if you are predisposed to overweight and obesity through genetics, genes do not act independently. They may also require certain behaviors such as overeating or low physical activity to be triggered.

It's quite possible that losing weight is more difficult for you than for your best friend. You can't change your genes, but you still have to ask yourself, *Have I done everything I can to manage my weight? Do I eat a healthy, balanced diet? Am I physically active? Do I engage in behaviors that may impact my weight, such as emotional eating or crash dieting? Have I examined the behaviors passed down to me from my parents, grandparents, aunts, and uncles and how they've affected my weight over the years? Is it really just a case of bad genes?*

Researchers point to the upsurge in overweight and obesity in this country as proof that genetics certainly can't be blamed for it. Instead, the blame goes to poor diet and an increasingly sedentary lifestyle for most Americans. The good news: these are all areas you can manipulate (unlike your genes) and work to change.

I've been waiting for the Fat Reaper my whole life. In kindergarten, I actually put my head down on my desk in embarrassment when my mother came to school with cupcakes. Everyone could see I had a fat mother. From a very early age, I expected to grow up and get fat because that was how your life progressed as a female: you got married, you had kids, and you got fat, just like my mother and my grandmother.

Even on my wedding day, I felt doomed to obesity. One of my husband's friends videotaped the ceremony. He was taping everything as though it were a journalistic event. Unfortunately, he captured one of the groomsmen telling my husband-to-be, "You've seen the mother, you've seen the grandmother … it's only a matter of time before Meredith looks like them." My husband made his friend erase the tape, but I heard about it anyway, and I was angry. But then I told myself he was just saying what everyone else at the wedding was thinking. Even on that happy day I felt doomed to be fat.

I had my children. After my son was born, I lost most of the weight I'd gained. Then my daughter was born in early 2001, and 6 weeks after her birth I still weighed 135 pounds, which is about 10 or 15 pounds more than I normally weigh at 5'6". Everyone kept telling me how great I looked, but I didn't like having that extra weight. I didn't look like me; I didn't *feel* like me. I was letting myself indulge in foods, which is something I'd never done before. I realized there was a lot of pressure from other people to give up on myself now that I was a mother. But I rebelled. In the fall of 2002, I made the decision that it was absolutely unacceptable for me to carry this extra weight, and I lost it. If you believe something is unacceptable, you won't do it.

I have a 5-pound comfort range. If I'm at the upper end of the range, I tell my husband, "I'm at maximum density," so I won't have pizza with the rest of the family. I have something else instead and maybe run an extra mile. I don't diet, but I watch everything I eat so that I can indulge once in a while. It means if I really want a Milano cookie, I can have one, but I certainly won't do that every day. I know genetics are stacked against me; if you tell me obesity is a disease, you put me at risk. I have to believe my weight is a choice that rests with me. —*Meredith, 36, New Jersey*

What Do Age, Sex, and Ethnicity Have to Do with It?

They're common-enough scenarios:

- A 55-year-old woman who has always carried extra weight in her hips and thighs notices that more fat is settling around her belly after menopause. In fact, her husband's developing a belly, too.

- A husband and wife join the same commercial weight-loss program. The wife watches everything that goes into her mouth and never skips workouts. The husband, on the other hand, still eats dessert and skips gym visits because of his work schedule. She's furious when she finds out he's lost more than she has in 6 months. "It's because you're a man, and men always lose weight easier!" she fumes.

- A doctor tells his patient he's concerned about his weight gain and blood sugar levels because he's a Latino. The patient is surprised to learn he's more at risk for developing serious complications from type 2 diabetes than members of other racial groups.

Like genetics, age, sex, and ethnicity play a part in the obesity puzzle. You lose muscle as you age, and fat starts to account for a greater percentage of your body mass. Less muscle mass means a slower metabolism, which means you don't need as many calories as you did when you were younger. That's why many trim, fit people are shocked when they notice a few extra pounds on the scales at an annual exam. They haven't changed anything in their diet or exercise regime, but that's precisely why they've gained. They may need to boost their energy output and decrease their food intake to maintain the weight they've held in the past. Moreover, as you age, you tend to slow down physically, which also contributes to weight gain.

Women get a double whammy. Men, by nature, have more muscle mass than women, so they have faster metabolisms. This is why your husband or boyfriend can eat more and exercise less and have no problems maintaining weight, whereas wives and girlfriends have to struggle and sweat to maintain theirs. Women also tend to put on weight after pregnancy. Research shows the average woman adds 4 to 6 pounds to her prepregnancy weight, and some researchers wonder if this, in some way, contributes to overweight and obesity in women. Then there's menopause. Decreasing levels of estrogen, a female sex hormone, is partly to blame for increased body fat, especially in the belly area.

There's also a racial and ethnic link to overweight and obesity. The American Obesity Association reports that overweight and obesity in the United States occur at higher rates for African Americans and Hispanics than they do for Caucasians. An African American female, for example, is two to three times more likely to be obese than a Caucasian female, which makes overweight and obesity significant health problems for this group. People who have a low socioeconomic status within minority populations are particularly at risk for overweight and obesity—especially women. Researchers suspect cultural factors that influence dietary and exercise behaviors play a major role in the development of excess weight in minority groups.

Psychological Factors On top of all the physical reasons why you tend to put on weight, you have to consider the dozens of psychological factors that work with your biology to prevent you from losing weight.

Emotional eating tops the list. If you've ever reached for a bag of cookies when you're feeling bored, or found that you gained weight during a particularly stressful time at work, you're well acquainted with emotional eating. Some of us eat because we've learned to associate food or eating with emotional comfort. Food becomes our best friend, our savior. And when it comes time to diet, it's difficult for most of us to turn our backs on our best friend.

Another challenge with emotional eating is that it's not something you can "cure" through willpower or dieting. The reasons why you eat when you're bored, angry, stressed, or even happy are triggered by chemical firestorms in your brain that occur in response to certain emotions. To "fix" the chemistry, you eat. And when you eat, your brain produces the chemicals that make you feel better. Basically, emotional eating becomes an addiction, and addictions are tough to break. Only when you understand why you eat when you're bored or anxious or happy can you accept new ways to soothe yourself—and manage brain chemistry—without food.

> ### PsychSpeak
>
> **Emotional eating** is characterized by excessive eating in the presence of anger, boredom, sadness, or even happiness.

All-or-nothing thinking is very common with dieters. It goes something like this:

You stick with your diet all week and then "blow it" with an extra slice of pizza after work on Friday. That's it. Your diet is ruined. On Saturday, you end up eating a whole pizza by yourself for lunch.

Or:

You decide you're going to lose 50 pounds by May 1. When you step on the scale on May 1, you've lost "only" 35 pounds. Rather than pat yourself on the back for losing the 35 pounds or checking your food diary to see what could be improved, you curse yourself for being a failure. You give up, and within a few months you've regained the 35 pounds—and then some.

All-or-nothing thinking is thinking in black and white. There's no gray, no middle ground. And when you only see your diet in black and white, you end up disappointed because diets, just like life, have a lot of gray areas.

Poor body image can lead to overweight and obesity. If you tell yourself you're fat, ugly, and worthless, you'll treat yourself like a fat person who's ugly and worthless. You'll eat foods that aren't good choices for you, and you won't take care of your health and appearance. Because you're unable to recognize much good in your appearance, it's hard for you to appreciate any positive changes you make in your diet or exercise program. Even if you do lose a few pounds, you may stand in a mirror, pinch your stomach, and tell yourself, *Yeah, but look at these rolls. Ugh.* Not very motivating, is it?

Tied into poor body image are the *media influences* that bombard us each day. From the constant barrage of fast-food commercials telling us "I'm lovin' it" (McDonald's) or that "we're the Pepsi generation," to the endless parade of celebrities who are impossibly thin and airbrushed to perfection, we struggle to remain fit in a world created by advertisers, corporations, publicists, and magazines. We succumb to the call of fast food while feeling depressed that we don't have Demi's toned tummy or Beyoncé's butt.

GET PSYCHED

"Even I don't wake up looking like Cindy Crawford."
–*Supermodel Cindy Crawford*

Our *values and beliefs* also play some role in our weight. If you value health and fitness, you stand a greater chance of avoiding obesity. On the other hand, someone who believes all family occasions must be celebrated with food is more likely to struggle with overweight and obesity. Why? Because not to engage in this behavior goes against what they hold dear—family, food, and love.

Only by examining their values and beliefs closely, and making a conscious decision to reframe them in a way that supports weight loss as well as what they value, will real change take place.

Other complex psychological factors contribute to overweight and obesity as well. Some people eat in response to a trauma, such as a sexual assault, a debilitating accident, or a loss of a close friend or family member. Rather than turn to alcohol or drugs to ease their pain, they turn to food. Other people turn to food when they quit smoking or stop using drugs. Roughly 80 percent of cigarette smokers, for example, gain weight when they quit their habit.

> ## GET PSYCHED
>
> "I've always believed that becoming overweight was not an option for me. If you ask me what I'd do if I hit 200 pounds, my answer would be I would *never* weigh 200 pounds, because I just wouldn't let my weight get that high. I do what I have to do to stay at my comfortable weight, around 180." *–John, 65, Bethel, Vermont*

Or maybe people around you actually encourage you to remain overweight or obese. You may have a spouse who regularly tells you, "I like you just the way you are." That can be a nice thing to hear if you only have a few pounds to lose or you're moderately overweight, but if you're severely obese and unhealthy, you have to wonder if your partner is encouraging you to continue living in this condition for other reasons. Could she be nervous that you'll lose weight and leave her? Is he afraid he'll lose his eating partner and be forced to examine his own relationship with food and overweight?

Brain Chemistry

Your weight is not only controlled by what you put in your body or how much you move during the day. It's also affected by an intricate dance of brain chemicals and hormones. As I've discussed, dozens of variables combine to affect your weight—from the genes you inherited from your parents, to your age, to how you cope with your emotions and treat your physical body. Combine these factors with the neurotransmitters, peptides, and hormones in your brain, and you can begin to understand how your brain has a great deal of control over your weight—from how and when you feel hunger and which foods you crave, to your body's ability and maybe even desire to lose weight.

Neuropeptide Y and Galanin Sarah F. Leibowitz, Ph.D., an adjunct associate professor in the Laboratory of Behavioral Neuroscience at The Rockefeller University in New York, studies behavioral processes of eating and physiological processes of metabolism and fat storage. Through studies with rats and mice, she has linked two neuropeptides called neuropeptide Y and galanin—both produced in the hypothalamus region of the brain—to what and when we eat, the hormones we secrete, and what we weigh on the scale. What's even more interesting is that every biological system responds to neurochemicals differently, depending on environmental and genetic factors. That is to say, your brain will have a slightly different reaction than your sister's brain when you share the same candy bar.

Neuropeptide Y has many complex effects on the body, from appetite control and sexual function, to circadian rhythms and stress and anxiety responses. It has also been linked to the regulation of feeding behavior. Upon awakening, do you reach for a Continental-style breakfast of toast, jam, coffee, and orange juice? If so, you can give neuropeptide Y the credit, as it's most active in the morning when you need a carbohydrate boost after a night's fast. Production of neuropeptide Y slows during the day, and another neuropeptide, galanin, revs up. Among other central nervous system actions, galanin affects your appetite for fats, which means later that evening you may find yourself hungry for a bowl of ice cream. Unfortunately, as Leibowitz suggests in a January/February 1993 article in *Psychology Today,* when you eat something fatty enough early in the day, it may generate more of this neurochemical to make you crave more fat that evening.

Neuropeptide Y and galanin production are sensitive to hormones. Leibowitz's research has shown cortisol, a hormone the body produces during stressful situations, coaxes the brain to produce more neuropeptide Y, which prompts a desire for carbohydrates. When the need for carbohydrates is satisfied by the release of another neurotransmitter, serotonin, the stress generated by biochemistry vanishes. This explains why you feel so much better after eating bread, cookies, or candy.

Galanin, on the other hand, is sensitive to the hormone estrogen. Leibowitz notes that children have little appetite for fat, preferring carbohydrates to fuel their energy. When girls hit puberty, their estrogen levels rise, which stimulates production of galanin in the brain. Their tastes change, and they're triggered to eat more fats, which they also need for sexual maturation.

Change Brain Chemistry to Lose Weight? In her research, Leibowitz has found that animals, like people, have individual preferences for nutrients, which, in turn, affect differences in feeding patterns. Nutrient preferences fall into three categories. Fifty percent of the population is biologically primed for a diet made up of approximately 60 percent carbohydrate, with 30 percent of calories coming from fat. Carbohydrate-driven subjects also tend to consume smaller, more-frequent meals and weigh significantly less than their peers.

GET PSYCHED

"The question is, can we find some specific dietary situation, different foods at different times, that might help us to reduce neuro-peptide activity without depriving ourselves? The whole point is, we can't deprive ourselves. But if we know that what we eat and when we eat it affect the production of neuropeptides, we can modulate what we eat and work the appetite so that we can get a new routine in."
—Sarah F. Leibowitz, Ph.D., adjunct associate professor, The Rockefeller University's Laboratory of Behavioral Neuroscience, quoted in Psychology Today, *January/February 1993*

Thirty percent of people and animals are biologically primed for a fat-based diet. These subjects consume the most calories, weigh the most, and tend to be affected by food cravings, especially at night. A biological preference for a protein-based diet seems to affect only a small number of subjects.

What does this mean for people who want or need to lose weight? Leibowitz's research seems to indicate diets based on re-striction of nutrients don't work. She claims that people need to understand the role brain chemistry plays in their weight and re-tune how it works. For example, don't skip meals. When you skip meals, you disrupt your brain's natural ebb and flow of neurochemicals, which, in turn, wreaks havoc on your appetite, your cravings, and your weight. When you deny your body the food it wants by starving it, your systems respond by producing more neurochemicals, which produces an even stronger drive to eat.

What You Can Do

Overweight and obesity are health conditions plaguing the majority of Americans. Maybe you're one of them. Sometimes experts make losing weight sound as simple as eating less and moving more, and in some respect, that's true. However, every American is a complex, highly individual biological system. Your body—and brain—has unique preferences and reactions to foods, dieting, and weight.

☐ Understand that overweight and obesity usually have many causes—causes you can work on and change.

☐ Examine the factors that may be influencing your own overweight and obesity. How much of a role do you think heredity has with your weight? How have your environment, behavior, socioeconomic status, age, sex, and race played a part?

☐ Observe how you think about such concepts as overweight, obesity, health, athleticism, and physical attractiveness.

☐ Make a list of all the reasons why weight loss would benefit you. Get as detailed as you can, and don't hold back. If you get excited about the thought of fitting into a pair of jeans you haven't worn in 10 years, that's a reason to hold on to.

☐ Ask yourself what you've been blaming for your weight gain. Do you blame your genes? Do you tell yourself you have no willpower? How much control do you think you have over your weight?

☐ Question how your unique brain chemistry affects your eating habits. Can you pick out any patterns that may be chemical-driven?

The Allure of the Quick Fix

I t's second nature for some Americans to want whatever's wrong in their lives fixed easily and fixed *now*. As a nation, we're used to getting things quickly—from our express mail to our fast food. Our expectations extend to diets and weight loss, and unfortunately, there's no shortage of people or companies around us offering a fast fix for our weight problems—for the low, low price of $29.99 a bottle!

Such companies take this knowledge and craft compelling sales messages that get us reaching for our wallets. The American Obesity Association estimates Americans spend $30 billion a year on diet sodas, diet foods, over-the-counter (OTC) diet pills and products, books, videos, weight-loss programs, and fitness memberships. With 45 million people attempting to lose weight at any given time, it's a great opportunity to offer fast results in return for a fast buck.

As a dieter and a consumer, you don't have to be a victim. You may have been attracted to quick fixes in the past and now realize they don't work for weight loss. On the other hand, you may still occasionally fall captive to the promise of an easy ride.

In this chapter, you learn why there's no easy fix for weight loss and good health.

In fact, what successful weight loss comes down to, for most people, isn't the diet itself but the *dieter*. And the real fix often costs far less than anything you can buy in a bottle.

Defining a Diet Quick Fix

A *quick fix* is a product, diet, or program that promises a short-term solution to a long-term problem. The following could be ads for quick fixes:

> *Our groundbreaking weight-loss pill will let you lose weight while you sleep!*
>
> *On the Santa Monica Grapefruit Diet, you'll never go hungry—and you'll lose weight like you've never lost before!*
>
> *Sign up today, and lose 5 pounds by next weekend!*

When you study quick-fix messages such as these, something becomes clear: there's no mention of any work on your part. The most effort you have to expend with the weight-loss pill is to go to bed. With the grapefruit diet, you don't even have to go to bed. And the third, well, it looks like you can just pay up and the pounds come off!

What's the Appeal? There's a good reason why you're not seeing any mention of work and effort for weight loss in these claims. Some diet marketers know the last thing millions of overweight Americans want to hear is that losing weight takes work and takes time. A message like that isn't sexy, and it doesn't sell books, shakes, and diet plans. As long as Americans continue to wear their blinders, these marketers have an easy—and profitable—market.

Sarah H., 41, of Baltimore, Maryland, agrees that dieters often hone in on the fast-fix or the surefire solution for weight loss, even when it's not presented in an advertisement. When people started noticing her 80-pound weight loss, she said they started peppering her with questions, eager for "the secret" to her loss.

"When I told them what 'the secret' was—cutting calories, measuring portions, and exercising hard—most people looked bored," she says.

And that's precisely it. Weight loss is basically a boring undertaking. It makes sense that advertisers want weight loss to look sexy, exciting, and easy. They know the truth is yawn-inspiring.

When Wishful Thinking Hurts Dieters know losing weight is boring, too, which leads us to wish our circumstances were otherwise. Most people who've engaged in chronic dieting at some point have engaged in wishful thinking. Robert Todd Carroll, in his book, *The Skeptic's Dictionary,* defines wishful thinking as "interpreting facts, reports, events, perceptions, etc., according to what one would like to be the case rather than according to the actual evidence."

With dieting, wishful thinking might go something like this:

> *Maybe this TV diet is different from all the others I've ordered.*
>
> *I know it makes no sense to drink only grapefruit juice for a week, but maybe I really can lose 5 pounds doing it.*
>
> *I'm not really good at showing up for meetings, but this time I won't skip any.*

If you're ever tempted by a diet, program, or product that sounds too good to be true or runs counter to how you typically behave in a diet, you can be sure that you're engaging in a bit of wishful thinking. Too much wishful thinking and you run the risk of jumping from diet to diet, hoping "this time will be different."

Before buying into wishful thinking, ask yourself some questions along these lines:

> *What hard evidence do I have that this television diet will be different from the others I've ordered?*
>
> *If something makes no sense to me, why am I willing to buy into it now, without investigating the claim further?*
>
> *In what ways have I changed that makes me think I won't skip meetings?*

You can ask yourself literally dozens of questions to get around wishful thinking so you can come to a rational, thoughtful decision about your next step.

Desperate Detours

Desperation leads some dieters to jump on the quick-fix bandwagon. It can be as simple as wanting to fit into a certain outfit within the next couple weeks, or more complex, such as struggling to lose weight to keep a spouse or partner. And some less-than-honorable marketers are very good at preying on the fears and emotions of people who are feeling desperate about their weight.

If you're at a point where you're feeling desperate about losing weight, step back for a moment. Desperation can be a good motivator, but it can also lead you to leaping without thinking. Chances are, any desperate attempt you make to lose weight will quickly leave you feeling more desperate. Better to take a deep breath and accept that a reasonable approach to weight loss will bring you more long-term benefits.

26

you're not alone

Maria, 38, grew up in a family that loved to eat. "Both my parents were from Mexico, and food was always important to them," she says. "My mother liked to cook, and my father liked to eat. Food was always the center of attention in my family."

Maria says she was "solid" growing up. "In high school, I weighed around 115 pounds (at 5'1"), and I thought that was fat," she says. She started skipping meals as a way to control her weight, and she also took up smoking after she heard it would curb her appetite.

At 19, Maria married her high school sweetheart; at 20, she had her first child without any complications. Four months after giving birth, she got pregnant with her second son. This pregnancy wasn't so easy. She ended up developing gestational diabetes. After her son's birth, Maria says she gave up ever thinking she'd be thin.

"I wasn't even 25, but my body felt worn out," she says. "It was just easier for me to sit around and eat." As the pounds added up, she says she would occasionally go on a diet, but nothing ever stuck. "It was more of the skipping meals and fasting, and I would only go back to eating more."

Maria found out she was pregnant again in her late 20s. "My husband and I were having marriage problems," she says, "and we both hoped a baby might help." This pregnancy almost killed her. Again, she developed gestational diabetes, and her daughter ended up being delivered by C-section, nearly 4 weeks premature.

Maria's recovery was slow, hampered by the fact that she had put on so much weight in 10 years. Maria was horrified when her doctor said her BMI was 35, which made her obese, and that she should lose weight. "I went home and cried because that word [obese] sounded so awful."

Unfortunately, Maria says her doctor didn't tell her *how* to lose the weight, so she started trying everything: ephedra, Atkins, weight-loss teas, and more. "If it said 'lose weight,' I bought it," she says. She also checked out stacks of diet books from the library. "My sons would say, 'Okay, Mom, what diet is it this week?' and roll their eyes."

"Even though I didn't go to college, I'm a smart person and knew a lot of stuff I was trying wasn't going to work," she says. "But I just kept hoping."

A friend introduced to her to a faith-based weight-loss program at her church in 2001, and that's where Maria says her thinking shifted. "It really was like having a religious experience," she says. "I finally felt a sense of relief that the crazy stuff was over." Maria began making simple changes: she stopped eating fast food or anything fried, she purchased a scale and portioned meals, and she added more fresh fruits and vegetables to her diet. Her husband bought her a treadmill so she could walk while watching her favorite soap operas. By the summer of 2002, Maria weighed 135 pounds—down from about 185 pounds—and her borderline high blood sugar had stabilized. She also quit her 20-year smoking habit while continuing to lose weight.

"I'd like to get down to 115 pounds," she says, "but I'm not willing to do anything crazy to get there. If I stay the weight I am for the rest of my life, I will be happy because I'm doing everything I can to be healthy. The rest is in God's hands."

Deciphering Dubious Claims

The Federal Trade Commission (FTC) has stepped up its efforts to watchdog unscrupulous diet marketers, but still, consumers are getting taken every day. While the agency continues to go after companies that create deceptive weight-loss messages, it's also educating consumers on claims that should make them stop and think.

WEB TALK: Check out the FTC's teaser site about bogus weight-loss claims at: ↑ wemarket4u.net/fatfoe/

Such claims include ...

- "Lose weight without diet or exercise!" You know if you're not seeing any mention of work or effort, the product is probably worthless. Maintainable weight loss takes consistent effort.

- "Lose weight no matter how much you eat of your favorite foods!" This claim goes into the "too good to be true" category. Getting to a healthy weight is all about making sensible food choices and watching how much you eat.

- "Lose weight permanently! Never diet again!" Long-term weight loss is something you'll work on for the rest of your life, but don't let that discourage you. When you finally find the eating plan that works for you, you really won't have to diet again!

- "Block the absorption of fat, carbs, or calories!" There is simply no magic pill that can do all these things. If you want to eat carbs or fats, eat them in moderation. And the only way to prevent the absorption of calories is to not eat them.

- "Lose 30 pounds in 30 days!" Losing more than 1 or 2 pounds per week is unhealthy. Products that promise more weight loss than this should be approached cautiously or not at all.

- "Everybody will lose weight!" There is no one diet that works for everyone, it's as simple as that. Successful dieting comes down to finding the right combination of foods, exercise, and behavioral changes that works for you.

  WEB TALK: Does losing weight while eating everything you want sound too good to be true? Check out the FTC's Amazing Claims website at: www.ftc.gov/bcp/conline/edcams/waistline/

- "Lose weight with our miracle diet patch or cream!" When you see the word *miracle* in a diet claim, walk away quickly. You cannot lose weight by rubbing a cream on your skin or placing a patch anywhere on your body.

If something about a diet quick fix smells fishy to you, it probably is. Your best bet is to report any diet claims that sound suspicious to your state's attorney general's office, a local consumer protection bureau, or the Better Business Bureau.

"So-and-So Told Me …"

Dieters also get looped into quick fixes by talking to other dieters. This is how I got mixed up with ephedra when it was still on the market. I was talking to a fellow writer at a business meeting who had lost 30 or so pounds—and quickly—by taking an ephedra-based dietary supplement. Eager to get such quick results myself, I ran out and bought myself a bottle of the product she recommended without doing any research. I discontinued taking the product after a few days because it made my heart race, and only then did I start asking questions. Had I asked them earlier, I would have saved myself $30 when I learned this product could be lethal for people with heart conditions, like the one I have.

Your friends, family, and acquaintances can be good sources of diet information, but their anecdotal information should be taken with a grain of salt. Even the smartest people go about losing weight in ways that aren't so safe—taking up cigarette smoking, for example. Moreover, every person is different. Just because your sister lost 25 pounds easily on a low-carb diet doesn't mean you'll have the same experience.

Listen to what your friends, family, and acquaintances have to say. If what they say sounds sensible to you, bring it to your health-care professional for discussion.

It's Not the Diet—It's *You!*

What successful weight loss comes down to is *you*. Although the diet and exercise you choose certainly have some bearing on your weight loss, more often than not it's the behaviors, attitudes, and habits you apply to the program that matter. There is no combination of foods or a breakdown of carbs, proteins, and fats that doctors can claim lead to better weight loss. However, successful dieters and long-term weight loss maintainers practice certain behaviors and habits—and you can, too.

You own your own diet, bottom line. No hard-and-fast rules govern what works and what doesn't—and although you may be tempted to think that sounds like bad news, it isn't. It means with a bit of experimentation, you can design or modify a weight-loss program that's just right for your body, your lifestyle, your goals, and your personality. You won't be able to pick up a book and follow steps A, B, and C, but you probably will be more successful than you've ever been before in taking off your weight—and keeping it off.

GET PSYCHED

"Read articles about losing weight. You can get so many hints and new ideas. Just be sure you make them *your* ideas. Never stop thinking *I want to feel better, look better, be healthier*—all those things equal losing weight." *–Donna, New York, New York*

What You Can Do

Remember—if a diet or a weight-loss product sounds too good to be true, it usually is. Lasting weight loss comes through sound decisions and consistent actions that spring from them—they don't come out of a bottle. Dieting is a daily effort, one with no shortcuts.

- ☐ Remain skeptical of diet claims. Anything that makes weight loss sound easy or effortless is usually not worth a second look.

- ☐ Whenever you're considering a weight-loss product or program, try to find out whether any clinical studies have been done on it and what the results are.

- ☐ Gather information on diets and weight loss from friends, family, and acquaintances, but remember this is just anecdotal evidence, not proof. Do your own research.

31

☐ If you suspect you've been taken by a product claim, file a report with the FTC at www.ftc.gov or by calling 1-877-FTC-HELP (1-877-382-4357; toll free); TTY: 1-866-653-4261.

☐ Keep in mind the actual diet you choose will be less responsible for your weight loss than you think. What lasting weight loss comes down to is you and how you think and behave over time.

Success Psychology

Only 5 percent of dieters are successful at losing weight and keeping it off. That means 95 percent of Americans who lose weight won't be able to keep it off. In consumer literature, this is the not-so-inspiring weight-loss success rate thrown at us. Whenever you hear these figures, you may think, *Why even bother trying? The odds are stacked against me*, and reach for another cookie or skip a workout.

However, a May 25, 1999 *New York Times* article questioned this dismal dieting success rate. The article's author, Jane Fritsch, talked to leading weight-control researchers around the country to find out where the 5 percent figure came from. She discovered it was from a clinical study conducted on 100 obese subjects at a New York weight-loss clinic in the 1950s. The subjects were given a standard diet without any support or attempts at behavior modification and told to report back on their successes. Given the lack of resources the study's subjects had, a 5 percent success rate actually sounds pretty good!

Researchers today say they have no firm percentage on the number of successful dieters. The number could be lower than 5 percent, but it also could be much higher, because resources available to dieters have greatly improved in the 40 or so years since the study was conducted. Moreover, it's difficult to come up with a firm percentage because not everyone joins a research study to lose weight—most people tend to go on diets from the comfort of their homes. Vast numbers of Americans lose weight—and keep it off—by making diet and exercise changes and learning weight-control skills without any clinical supervision.

This said, researchers are getting closer to finding out why some people are more successful at losing weight than others by studying the exciting data available to them. They're also studying how change occurs in populations, which may make it easier to develop public health programs to combat overweight and obesity in the future.

Why We Decide to Change

One way researchers are learning more about weight-loss success is through a data repository called the National Weight Control Registry (NWCR), which has compiled statistics on more than 4,000 people who've lost 30 pounds or more and kept it off for upward of 1 year. The NWCR is not a study, but purely a voluntary database of successful dieters who have shared details about what helped them succeed at weight loss.

Some interesting information has come out of the data. A whopping 91 percent of registrants had tried to lose weight before their successful try, often dozens of times. However, researchers found during the successful try, a little more than 80 percent of registrants increased their exercise; 63 percent were stricter with their diets; and 85 percent reported improvements in their health, quality of life, energy levels, mobility, moods, and levels of confidence. Moreover, change wasn't

GET PSYCHED

"Success is not down the road. It can be precisely where you are on the road, right now, today."
–Victoria Moran in Fit from Within

easy for them. Around 40 percent said losing weight was hard, 30 percent said it was moderately hard, and only 25 percent said it was easy.

Most registrants didn't decide to lose weight because it was something they thought they should do. A majority (77 percent) said a medical or emotional event triggered their weight loss.

Health Triggers   The NWCR says 32 percent of people decided to lose weight because of a health condition. Often the development of a significant health problem associated with overweight or obesity causes people to say, "That's it! The weight's coming off."

Sometimes it takes a significant wake-up call to get people to change. They may have realized for years that they had to do something about their weight but avoided taking action. Suddenly it's not a matter of when they'll take action, but how fast they can take it.

A Personal Trigger   Other people are successful at losing weight after weathering a personal crisis, such as any of the following:

- The death of a family member or friend from an obesity-related disease or condition
- Marriage or divorce
- Having children
- Not liking the way they feel in their clothes or how they look in the mirror
- Suffering a blow to self-esteem, such as being told they're fat

you're not alone

The only time Bo McCoy of Capistrano Beach, California, left his house was to go to work as a seasonal tax preparer. At 626 pounds, it was difficult to get dressed in the morning, and keeping himself presentable was always a challenge. "I had to struggle to maintain a good public persona," he said. "When you're fat, you don't want to have enemies."

One co-worker began making derogatory comments about his weight and how he smelled, claiming that his presence was inappropriate for an office. Bo's co-workers suggested he confront this woman, and he did. Surprisingly, she didn't deny what she'd said. "It was rude in the way she said it," Bo recalls, "but she wasn't lying. I *did* struggle with body odor; at over 600 pounds, it was really hard to control."

Bo was embarrassed and felt debased by the confrontation. He went into the men's room where he could be by himself and began to weep. "I knew I'd gotten to a place where I was out of control." That day, he gave his notice.

He was upset for days, but finally a friend who'd had gastric bypass surgery asked Bo to lunch. She brought her before and after pictures and suggested he consider the surgery. That night, Bo began researching options on the Internet. He adopted a line from the movie *The Shawshank Redemption* as his personal motto: "Get busy living, or get busy dying." He got busy living. Six months later, he had the Roux-en-Y surgical procedure, and lost 200 pounds within 6 months after the surgery.

Bo did very little formal exercise the first year of his weight loss. Indeed, just being able to move around helped him increase his activity levels. After a year, he started walking, eventually getting up to a 1.5-mile walk.

Today, Bo weighs 245 pounds; he's lost about 385 pounds in almost 3 years. His life today is so radically different from the way it used to be, he doesn't know where to begin listing the changes. "Imagine having to wear a 400-pound suit for years and then being able to take it off, knowing you never have to wear it again. It's a life without boundaries." *(For more of Bo's amazing transformation, visit his website at www.72inches.com.)*

A Little of Both Sometimes people change because of a combination of health and personal reasons that converge at the right moment. This was certainly my case. My doctor had just finished telling me I was officially overweight and had high blood cholesterol, and I'd recently received a picture of myself in the mail that made me look like an out-of-shape, middle-aged woman. I didn't like it, so I decided to change.

Two successful weight-loss retainers interviewed for this book reported they'd gotten sick and lost a few pounds. Their poor health played a role in motivating their personal desire to lose weight. They saw the additional weight loss as a challenge.

Whether you're driven to change because of health problems or you're compelled to change because you don't recognize the person staring back at you in the mirror, remember that one reason isn't any more valid than another. What matters is that the desire is compelling enough for you to start looking for solutions.

Understanding the Stages of Change

James O. Prochaska, Ph.D., a psychologist at the University of Rhode Island in Kingston, has spent his professional life studying why and how people change. Prochaska, along with his colleagues, developed a theory that people have to go through certain stages before they make successful changes in their lives. His theories have proved so accurate that companies are using them for health programs that correctly target employees at differing levels of change. Prochaska believes that, to be effective, an appeal to someone who's on the verge of making a change will have to be different than for a person who's just contemplating change. Prochaska's five stages of change are:

Precontemplation. The person may not know they have a problem with their weight, and they may even deny having a weight problem. A precontemplator believes he doesn't have to change; the people around him should. For example, a husband complains his wife is always nagging him to lose weight, and he wishes she would just stop nagging. A person in this stage is resisting change;

they may even be demoralized. Prochaska believes that even precontemplators can progress toward change if they get the right message.

Contemplation. Contemplators notice they have a problem and they start thinking about how to change it and even come up with some solutions. However, they're not quite ready to take action. This stage can last for years. It's the stage in which dieters talk about losing weight and say they'll change "someday." They may eternally substitute thinking for action, which turns them into a chronic contemplator. When people reach the end of this stage, they start thinking more about the solution rather than the problem, and the future rather than the past.

Preparation. People in the preparation stage are almost ready to take action. They're setting goals and making final adjustments to their plans. At this point, they may feel a little ambivalent about losing weight, yet they've instituted some small changes already—drinking more water during the day, for example, or beginning to walk after dinner.

Action. Showtime! This is where more overt change takes place. People in this stage are doing something to lose the weight, and others are noticing. Prochaska says this is where people, even professionals, can get sidetracked from their goal because they equate action with change, whereas change also includes the stages that come *before* and *after* action.

Maintenance. This is where changers work to maintain the gains they've made and figure out what they have to do to prevent relapse. "Change doesn't end with action," Prochaska writes in *Changing for Good*. It's a long, ongoing process, especially with long-term weight loss. However, at this stage, people are usually confident that they'll be able to maintain the change for a lifetime.

What habit should I work on first—eating a better diet or starting an exercise program? Or can I work on both habits at the same time?

"The old wisdom was to change one thing at a time, because you shouldn't take too much action at once," says James O. Prochaska, Ph.D., author of *Changing for Good.* But it's fine to work on more than one behavioral change at once if you're ready to take action on each one of them. On the other hand, if you're ready to work on your diet but not so ready to start an exercise program, that's okay, too. Prochaska points out that if you succeed in changing that first behavior (the healthy eating), you're three times more likely to succeed at changing the second behavior (exercising more). When you change one behavior (eating less), the second behavior you change (exercising more) will catch up to that first change with time.

In a perfect world, people move smoothly from stage to stage, eventually making the change they want. But usually that's not what happens. People tend to move back and forth among stages, often for years, before they move on to another stage. Returning to a previous stage of change, or relapse, tends to happen with weight loss, especially when dieters have reached the action or maintenance stages of change. Yet few people tend to return to the first stage of change, precontemplation. The majority of people go back to contemplation or preparation, and, as with quitting smoking, actually become more likely to achieve change with future attempts.

If dieters do relapse, Prochaska's advice is to look over what they did right on the

GET PSYCHED

"Every time I come back to improve my health, I've learned something from the last time." *–Donna, New York, New York*

diet and analyze mistakes made so future efforts at change have a roadmap. "See the earlier attempt as a learning experience, not a failure," he says.

My life is kind of stressful right now. Should I try to change my eating behaviors when life gets less stressed, or go for it now?

Experts (as well as dieters) are divided on the subject of change readiness. Some believe readiness needs to be assessed and that change should be attempted when conditions are "right"–for example, no major life changes on the horizon or the dieter seems motivated to change.

However, others think change can and should be attempted when conditions aren't perfect. "People can make changes when their motivation is down," says Elena Ramirez, Ph.D., director of the Weight Control Clinic at the University of Vermont. "There are very few people who are ever at the right place to make changes. My thought is that if you're clinically overweight, you need to start something." She points out that even if the person isn't fully motivated to lose weight but she simply doesn't gain weight over her 12-week program, it can be a good thing. Another point: all dieters have to learn how to manage their weight during stressful times, such as during job changes or over the holidays. In Ramirez's view, there's no time like the present to learn how.

What Predicts Success?

First, the bad news: there's no easy formula for weight-loss success. Think about it. Have you ever met someone who lost a tremendous amount of weight and then asked what worked for him? He tells you, "Well, I eat a high-protein diet, I run two miles at 5 A.M. before work, I never eat after 6 P.M., and I don't snack between meals." That may be a surefire success plan for him, but if you're not a high-protein kind of eater, you don't even know what 5 A.M. looks like, you can't imagine eating dinner before 8 P.M., and no snacks ... forget it!

What weight-loss success comes down to for most people is a combination of proven behaviors others have used along with their own personal preferences. For example, study after study shows people who eat breakfast in the morning have an easier time losing weight and keeping it off. But several of the successful dieters interviewed for this book told me they never ate breakfast. I'm not advising that you skip breakfast, but if eating breakfast is just something you can't do when you wake up, then work on changing another behavior that's not so difficult for you.

One thing diet companies are really good at is convincing customers that "this diet will be different." They pitch that the food plan or combinations of food they're touting are what have been standing between you and success. Quite frankly, the composition of the diet isn't what makes some dieters more successful than others; it almost always comes down to the behaviors they used with the diet, whether it was low-calorie, high-protein, or any of the dozens of other reasonable diets out there.

Successful dieters do tend to share certain qualities, however.

A Moderate Approach People who've managed to lose weight and keep it off report that what finally worked for them was a diet based on moderation. They may have spent a lifetime eating no carbs one week and no fat the next, but finally they discover, with a sense of relief, that moderation works for them.

Characteristics of this kind of thinking include ...

- Portion sizing. Some dieters literally weigh everything that goes into their mouths. This can be a highly effective way to "re-teach" yourself what a pat of butter or 4 ounces of chicken breast looks like. When Claire, a dieter from

Chicago, was learning how to manage cravings, her therapist asked her to buy all her favorite "crave" foods. Each day she was required to eat one serving of the food, weighing out a serving as specified on the container, no matter if she was craving it or not. "It totally rewired me," she says. "I no longer think of those foods as 'special.' They're just foods."

- No "bad" or "good" foods. This doesn't mean these dieters still eat everything. They may indeed be watching fat grams, but they'll eat a cookie now and then. But now, the cookie is the exception, not the rule.

- Monitoring hunger and satiety signals. This often takes dieters a long time to relearn, especially after a lifetime of overeating. But eventually, successful dieters become good at learning to eat only when they're hungry and to stop when they're not.

Health Versus Appearance Some people successfully lose weight based on a desire to "look good," but for most people, it becomes more important to "feel great." A woman may start out wanting to lose weight so she can fit into size 10 clothing again, but as the weight comes off, she starts noticing other benefits, such as lower blood cholesterol levels or a higher amount of energy.

Successful dieters usually have shifted their thinking from *I've got to lose weight*, to *I want to be healthy*. It may explain why a significant percentage of dieters decide to lose weight after learning about a health problem, such as severe hypertension or diabetes. They must change the way they look at food, because if they don't, it will kill them.

Attitude A successful dieter not only tends to be moderate in her eating, but also in her thinking. For example, someone who engages in "all-or-nothing" thinking is going to have a harder time finding success than someone who accepts that life is rarely black and white. It doesn't mean they're any less serious about their diet, but they realize perfection, especially in dieting, doesn't exist.

Some other attitude-adjustment traits include ...

- They do what they have to do. Successful dieters usually get to a point in their lives where they don't think; they just do. They get up and run before work because it's what they do. They watch portion size because it's what they do. They don't pay attention to how others are eating because that's not what *they* have to do to stay healthy.

- They've stopped playing the blame game. So they have a family history of overweight and obesity. They may have been obese themselves. But at some point they realize they've been letting genes dictate their behaviors, and they start changing what they can change, not what they can't.

- "If I can do it, you can do it." People who've successfully lost weight are usually enthusiastic about telling other people how they changed their lives. This kind of zeal generates a positive pressure on them to continue maintaining their new lifestyles.

What You Can Do

People can and *do* lose weight permanently, and so can you. Even if you've been on every diet there is and feel unsure of your chances of success this time, keep in mind that research shows most long-term changers have tried and failed—and tried and failed—before finding success.

☐ Forget what you've read or heard about the mere 5 percent of dieters who manage to lose their weight for good. The figure from this 45-year-old study is not applicable to successful dieters today.

☐ Talk to people close to you about what made them finally change a habit or addiction. If you know an ex-smoker, what made her quit? If your co-worker used to bite her nails, what triggered her to stop? You'll be surprised at what you learn.

☐ Assess where you are in the stages of change. Are you still unconvinced that you need to lose weight, or are you actively making plans to start your diet next Monday?

☐ Remember: lasting change can occur by taking small steps.

☐ Read books about people who've made amazing changes in their lives. The changes don't have to be weight-related, but the motivation for change or the process for change might inspire you.

☐ Understand that although you may have been on dozens of diets before, you have never been in the moment you're in now. You're a different person than you were during those other diets, and you're in different circumstances. This time can be different for you.

☐ Change is scary. Accept that as you try to change your habits, you will feel emotions such as doubt, anxiety, and ambivalence. Just don't give up.

Part 2

Weight Loss That Works for You

Now for the nitty-gritty. Count carbs or count calories? Eat like your ancestors, or dine as they do in the Mediterranean? In Part 2, you get an overview of the different ways to lose weight so you can pick a plan—or design your own—that works for you and your lifestyle.

Restriction Diets

I f you've ever tried to lose weight—whether a few pounds here and there, or a hundred pounds or more—you're probably well acquainted with the concept of restriction dieting. If you're on a restriction diet, you write down the calorie and carbohydrate count of everything that passes your lips. Most commercial weight-loss centers offer this kind of diet, where food is assigned "points" and you can eat only your allotted number of points each day.

Restriction diets follow a basic diet truth: you lose weight when you eat less. What has the experts—everyone from university researchers and government officials to dieticians and author M.D.s—at odds with each other is *what* you should eat less *of*. Less fat? The low-carb proponents claim reducing fat grams doesn't work because carbs make you fat. These experts point to the continuing rise of obesity levels in the United States when cutting dietary fat was all the rage. The experts who recommend watching fat intake, on the other hand, express serious concerns about the safety as well as the science behind a low-carb diet. They claim it encourages dieters to consume more unhealthy saturated fats to the neglect of the healthy carbohydrates found in fruits, vegetables, and whole grains. They also pooh-pooh the idea that carbs are solely responsible for the growing obesity problem in our country, and instead point to other factors, such as increased caloric intake, lack of exercise, and excess dietary fat.

There's also the million-dollar question experts (and dieters) would like to have answered once and for all: what kind of restriction plan is easiest for dieters to follow? The human body and psyche are programmed to rebel against restriction, which is why so many restrictive-type diet plans are abandoned before weight-loss goals are reached. How can dieters compete with a formidable opponent such as biology? And lastly, if you manage to stick to a restriction diet, what happens when you've reached your goal? Does biology rear its head and drive you to eat all the foods and calories you've been assiduously avoiding for months? And which restriction diet offers the best chance for maintaining weight after weight loss is achieved?

All these questions mean there's no "one-size-fits-all" restriction diet—and that's good news for dieters. Literally hundreds of diet plans are based on restriction, and what works wonders for one person may not be the best plan for her neighbor. If you're interested in a diet based on restriction, you may have to try a few to see which one best fits your needs. The upside is that with all the plans out there, you'll surely be able to find one you can follow, if not embrace.

What Are Restriction Diets?

A restriction diet limits the intake of calories, foods, and/or substances such as fats and carbohydrates to encourage weight loss. They're the most popular of weight-loss plans.

Restriction diets, sometimes called reducing diets, work on the principle that the human body requires a certain caloric intake each day to maintain weight and perform basic bodily functions. This number of calories is commonly referred to as the *basal metabolic rate (BMR)*.

Basic bodily functions include everything from breathing oxygen and digesting food to regulating body temperature. On top of that, your body needs additional calories to support daily activities. If you're not a very active person, your body won't need many additional calories, as opposed to someone who walks briskly for 45 minutes a day or who trains for an athletic event. However, when you increase your activity level, your body burns even more energy, which is precisely why exercise is a recommended component of weight-loss plans (see Chapter 9).

> **PsychSpeak**
>
> **Basal metabolic rate** or **BMR** is the number of calories you need per day to maintain bodily functions at your current weight.

You're probably beginning to see the picture. When you consume more calories than your body needs to maintain its current weight, those calories don't get burned off. Instead, your body converts them to fat and finds a place to store it—depots such as your thighs, hips, stomach, upper arms, and under your chin. Likewise, when you don't consume enough calories to support your current weight, your body has no choice but to start burning the excess body fat stored in your body's depots.

The goal of a safe, effective restriction diet is to force the body to burn through these fat stores at a controlled, even pace—no more than 2 pounds or 1 percent of body weight per week. What dieters have to watch out for are restriction plans that cause their bodies to lose weight *too* rapidly. A diet that promises followers they can drop 5 or 10 pounds in a week are simply unsafe. These "crash diets" (see Chapter 6) are usually too low in calories and/ or nutrients—and less of either does not equal better or more weight loss. At best, they force the body to lose water weight, and at worst, they cause serious short- and long-term damage to your health—everything from electrolyte imbalances leading to heart failure to bone-density loss. Too-rapid weight loss also causes the body to burn muscle mass, the one thing you *don't* want to lose when you're dieting. The more muscle you have, the faster and more efficient you become at burning off the real culprit—excess body fat.

The Pros and Cons of Restriction Diets

If losing weight were as simple as restricting food intake, we'd be all set. But there's something else at work, and unfortunately it works against the good intentions of dieters: our bodies are evolutionarily, biologically—and even psychologically—programmed to battle restriction.

While mankind has wrought all kinds of changes upon the world over tens of thousands of years, the world has wrought little change on the human body. Our bodies and our metabolic functions differ little from those of our ancient ancestors, who spent their lives hunting wild game and gathering foodstuffs from the land.

Our ancestors had to contend with the constant threat of droughts, famines, and seasonal changes to their food supplies. Evolution helped mankind adapt to these threats by making metabolic shifts within the body that helped the species survive these physically demanding events. A famine, for example, severely reduces the amount of food available to a society. While our ancestors struggled to survive on the minimal amounts of food available to them, their bodies adapted by slowing down their metabolisms to conserve energy and weight. When food supplies increased, their bodies didn't make an abrupt switch back to prefamine efficiency. As a self-protective measure, their metabolisms stayed slow to build up energy stores, a.k.a. body fat, in case of another famine.

Because seasonal changes, famines, and droughts are a regular occurrence, the human body has adapted to this feast-and-famine cycle. As humans advanced technologically, we learned better ways to survive these cycles of ups and downs. We learned how to plant crops and preserve foods for tough times. We developed snares, traps, nets, and guns to make hunting and fishing easier. Eventually we developed machines to do most of the back-breaking work of farming. Today, few of us have to rely on our own labor and wits to remain well fed. Machines and technology do most of the work for us. The only energy we burn is when we walk through the supermarket tossing what we need for dinner into a shopping cart.

Evolution's a slow process; our bodies haven't quite figured out that famine is something we can cope with through tech-nology. That means if you start consuming too few *calories,* your body goes through the same biochemical changes the ancient hunter/gatherers' bodies experienced during times of famine. Your metabolism slows down, and it becomes more difficult for you to lose weight. You become frustrated as well as hungry. The more you severely restrict those calories, the harder your body fights to hang onto fat. And over time, it becomes more difficult to lose the weight.

PsychSpeak

A **calorie** is a unit of heat equal to the energy it takes to raise the temperature of 1 gram water by 1 degree Celsius.

On top of this, you have to deal with psychological resistance to restriction. Our brains don't respond well to denial. Have you ever gone on a diet and told yourself, *I'm only going to eat 1,000 calories a day—not one calorie more?* First of all, a 1,000-calorie-a-day diet is going to put your body into feast-or-famine mode pretty quickly. You might last a few days or maybe a couple weeks on it, but soon your brain starts assisting biology. You start thinking about food, craving it even. It appears to you in your dreams. If you try not to think about food, your brain works even harder to get you to notice you're starving. Every fast-food ad swallows your attention, or you start salivating whenever you think of steak. Soon, you're chin-deep in a 5,000-calorie free-for-all. Your body and brain give each other a high-five and say, *Whew, glad we averted that famine. Better hold onto these calories for her next diet!*

So the key with a restriction diet is to figure out how to "trick" evolutionary biology and psychology to work with safe and healthful modern-day restriction plans. You have to reduce calories to the point where your body isn't triggered into thinking it's starving. And you have to eat foods that keep your brain from screaming, *I'm being denied!*

Counting Calories

Counting calories is the most basic restriction diet of all. It's not sexy, and it's not new—but when calorie counting is done correctly, it's one of the most effective ways to lose weight. It's also one of the more simple diet plans around. All you really need to do is track how many calories you take in each day. You can check calorie counts of certain foods by reading labels, and if no label exists, dozens of calorie-count books are on your local bookstore shelves, just waiting to help you. If you don't feel like buying a book, check out one of the many free calorie counters on the web. Some even allow you to track and store your calorie counts. You can even join weight-loss sites or buy software that make calorie-counting a breeze (see Chapter 8 for resources).

WEB TALK: Check out The Calorie Control Council's online calorie counter at:

www.caloriescount.org/cgi-bin/calorie_calculator.cgi

When you're counting calories, you're free to eat what you want as long as you don't exceed your target caloric intake for the day. The diet doesn't "forbid" any foods unless *you* decide they're forbidden. So if you want to eat your 1,400 allotted calories in the form of ice cream, you may do so and you'll still lose weight. However, you'll soon figure out that 1,400 calories of ice cream isn't enough ice cream to keep you going all day. Ice cream is calorie-dense, meaning 1 tablespoon of Ben and Jerry's New York Super Fudge Chunk will have more calories than, say, 1 tablespoon of plain, nonfat yogurt. You'll be able to eat a lot more of plain, nonfat yogurt by volume than you will of the Ben and Jerry's.

This is precisely why the most effective calorie-counting plans include nutrient-rich, low-calorie foods such as plain, nonfat yogurt that will keep you feeling satisfied.

The real trick to calorie-counting is figuring out how many calories *you* need every day to encourage safe, sensible weight loss. Depending on your sex, age, metabolism, and activity levels, your number is going to be different than your neighbor's. Experts recommend that females consume no less than 1,200 calories a day and males no less than 1,600 calories. Some diets go below these numbers, but only follow such diets under a doctor's supervision.

To start calorie-counting, first figure out your current BMR: multiply your weight (in pounds) by 10 if you're a woman, and by 11 if you're male.

> *Example:* If you're a 220-pound female, your current BMR to maintain basic bodily functions is 2,200 calories per day (220 × 10 = 2,200).

You also need calories above this number to help you perform daily activities such as walking, housework, and yard work.

Those additional calories are determined by your metabolism, age, sex, and activity level. A sedentary 50-year-old woman may only need a few extra calories above her BMR to maintain weight. A moderately active 25-year-old woman could need 30 to 50 percent more calories over her BMR. An extremely fit athletic male in his 30s could need 100 to 200 percent more calories over his BMR to maintain his current weight.

> *Example:* If you're a 250-pound male who's moderately active, your current BMR to support basic bodily functions plus additional activity can range from 3,575 calories to 4,125 calories per day [2,750 + (2,750 × 30%) = 3,575] or [2,750 + (2,750 × 50%) = 4,125].

"Wait," you're saying. "I want to *lose* weight, not maintain my current weight." In this case, you have to figure out the BMR for your target weight, along with how many additional calories you'll need to support your individual metabolism and activity needs.

Let's say you're a 220-pound female and you have a goal weight of 140 pounds. The BMR for your target weight is 1,400 calories per day (140 × 10 = 1,400). If you're moderately active, you'll need some additional calories, anywhere from 420 to 700 calories. You may have to adjust this number for your age, individual metabolism, and activity levels, but a good starting point is to set your calorie intake between 1,820 and 2,100 calories a day. If you continue to gain weight or your weight doesn't budge, reduce your calories by 5 or 10 percent until you start to achieve weight loss, no more than 2 pounds per week. If you start losing more than this, or 1 percent of your current body weight, increase the calories by 5 or 10 percent until your weight loss slows to a safe pace. Also, check your activity levels—you may be more or less active than you think. Increasing your activity level is going to boost your metabolism, which in turn will help you burn calories faster.

Too much math for you? Another way to determine your target caloric intake for the day is to multiply your current weight by 10. This will allow for a modest half-pound-per-week weight loss.

Commercial Programs

Commercial weight-loss programs are an attractive option for many people who want to lose weight. The three largest weight-loss franchises in the United States are Weight Watchers, Jenny Craig, and LA Weight Loss, and dozens of other programs exist as well, including NutriSystem, Diet Center, and Physicians Weight Loss Center, among others. Their biggest draw is that they offer structure to dieters who don't want to lose weight on their own. They hand you the instructions, guidelines, and support, and sometimes they even provide you with the food and supplements you'll need for their programs. You don't need to think up any food rules for yourself; they've already done that for you. You eat the foods they tell you to eat in the amounts they specify, you drink what they say you should, you swallow the nutritional supplements they often sell, and you're assured to lose weight. There are other draws to these programs.

- They're convenient. Just about every major city has a Weight Watchers center; and in church basements and community centers in small towns across the United States, you'll find Weight Watchers meetings. Other weight-loss centers can be found in strip malls and office buildings. Many companies even offer on-site centers for their employees. Too busy to drop by? You can join these programs online and get virtual guidance.

- They offer accountability. When you're trying to lose weight on your own, you're only accountable to yourself and the scale. But if you know you have to weigh in at a weekly meeting or share your food diary with a counselor, you might be more motivated to stick to your diet.

- They offer camaraderie. Dieting can be a lonely journey, and it's nice to talk to a counselor or other dieters who are walking the same path as you.

- They can be nutritionally sound. Doctors often recommend programs such as Weight Watchers and Jenny Craig to their overweight patients because these programs encourage members to lose weight sensibly—no more than 2 pounds per week on a balanced diet.

- They often have "real world" testimonials. Because so many dieters turn to these commercial weight-loss programs, chances are good you know someone who's been successful on one of them. Seeing the positive results yourself in someone you actually know can be a powerful incentive for you to join.

you're not alone

All my life I've been heavy. I came from a Greek home, where the rule was you licked your plate clean. I remember my mom buying me the Husky-sized jeans in the boys department in Sears. And I never exercised—are you kidding? Fat girls don't exercise! The older I got, the heavier I got. In 1992, I herniated some discs in my back. My doctor told me that if I lost some weight, it would relieve the pressure and pain in my back. So I signed up with Jenny Craig and lost 50 pounds.

Then I got married, had two children, and gained all the weight back, plus some. During my last pregnancy, I developed gestational diabetes. This time my doctor told me that by the time I was 45 or 50, I'd be full-blown diabetic. It scared me, but not enough. In 2002, my back went out again. Now my doctor was telling me I'd have to get surgery. Finally something clicked. I remember thinking, *How many times does someone have to tell me to lose weight? I've got to do something because I'm*

Is a commercial weight-loss program any more effective than, say, a weight-loss program you design yourself? Unfortunately, there's not a lot of scientific proof to back up media testimonials and advertising that claim the commercial programs are better. The authors of a research study published in 2005 in the *Annals of Internal Medicine* concluded that commercial weight-loss centers need to sponsor more controlled trials of their programs to provide scientific evidence of how effective they are at helping clients lose weight. Thomas Wadden and Adam Tsai at the University of Pennsylvania Health System looked for sponsored studies in which subjects were on the program for longer than 12 weeks and had their weight assessed after a year. The only commercial weight-loss center that met their criteria was Weight Watchers, which sponsored a controlled study showing that subjects lost about 5 percent of their starting weight over 3 to 6 months and kept off 3 percent after a year. There were no such studies conducted by Jenny Craig or LA Weight Loss, or any of the seven other programs they reviewed. The authors' intent wasn't to slam the commercial

going straight downhill. I decided to go back to Jenny Craig because I'd had success with the program before.

I need a lot of structure. I didn't want to spend a lot of time weighing food, counting calories, and figuring out portion sizes. Jenny Craig handed me the food, and I fit it into my life. The weight started coming off, 1 to 3 pounds a week, and I started to feel more confident. When I hit my goal weight in 2004, I was ready to learn how to do my own portion control and incorporate my own meals, which the program showed me how to do.

I was overweight for 36 years and used to wear a size 22. Today, I wear a size 6 and I exercise a half-hour with tapes every day. I can walk into the Gap with my 16-year-old nieces and find clothes I can wear. My back doesn't hurt me anymore, and my doctor is happy with my blood sugar levels. I've done everything in my power to get my health back, and I'm the healthiest I've ever been in my life. —*Chris S., 37, Oceanside, New York*

weight-loss industry. Instead, they hoped their findings would spur them to conduct more controlled trials of their programs so consumers could have more facts and less hearsay about the programs' effectiveness. In fact, after Wadden and Tsai's report was published, Jenny Craig announced it was beginning a controlled trial of its program in the coming months.

Beyond the fact that it's extremely difficult, if not impossible, for prospective members to get science to back up success rates, keep in mind the following things when evaluating commercial weight-loss centers:

- The fees for commercial weight-loss programs can be steep. They'll entice you with special deals, such as no sign-up fees or 6 weeks for $36. But many programs require extra money for weekly meetings, prepackaged foods, and supplements.

- They often hire counselors who have no formal qualifications beyond the company's own training. They may be experienced in their own weight loss and can certainly be a mentor to members, but they may not be providing the most accurate, scientific information about nutrition, weight loss, psychology, and/or exercise.

- They have high drop-out rates, just as do-it-yourself diets do. Although you may initially feel the program gives you some accountability, it's the middle part of the journey where you need to keep your motivation up. You must be as committed to a commercial program as an individual program, because success still comes down to you!

The weight loss center I visited said I must buy all their supplements if I want to join their program. They were vague about how the supplements work, but they wanted me to sign up right away. What else should I ask about the program?

Before investing in a commercial diet program, the U.S. Federal Trade Commission (FTC) recommends you ask the following questions:

- What are the health risks with this program?
- What data can you show me that proves your program actually works?
- Do customers keep off the weight after they leave your diet program?
- What are the costs for membership, weekly fees, food, supplements, maintenance, and counseling? What's the payment schedule? Are any costs covered under health insurance? Do you give refunds?
- Do you have a maintenance program? Is it part of the package, or does it cost extra?
- What kind of professional supervision is provided? What are the credentials of these professionals?
- What are the program's requirements? Are there special menus or foods, counseling visits, or exercise plans?

If the answers you receive don't make sense to you, don't sign up! Investigate the program through your local Better Business Bureau or state attorney general's office before parting with your money—and possibly your health.

Carbohydrate Restriction

You can't walk through a grocery store these days without seeing a food product or packaging marked "low-carb" or "carb-friendly" or pick up a restaurant menu where the *net carbs* are indicated next to the meal's price. Indeed, low-carb mania has propelled

PsychSpeak

Net carbs are a food's total carbohydrates minus fiber, glycerin, and sugar alcohols. It is a marketing phrase used to highlight a lower carb count, not a government or scientific term. Net carbs allow for the fact that fiber, glycerin, and sugar alcohols don't raise blood sugars like other carbs. But sugar alcohols may raise blood sugar, and they certainly do add calories.

food marketers and farmers to develop low-carb versions of verboten foods such as breads, pastas—even spuds! A farming cooperative in Florida has developed a potato that has 70 percent of the carbs found in a Russet potato.

The theory behind carbohydrate-restriction diets is pretty simple: proponents say when you cut back on carb-rich foods such as breads, pastas, sugars, vegetables, and fruits, your body turns to burning fat, rather than carbs, for energy. Most researchers won't disagree that Americans eat too many empty carbs—white breads, white rice, and sugar, for example. What they do find troubling about carb-restriction diets is that they pull dieters away from the good carbohydrates—whole-grain breads rich in fiber and vitamins, or fiber-rich legumes loaded with cancer-fighting nutrients. And let's face it—most Americans haven't been getting fatter from eating the carbs found in vegetables and whole grains.

Does carb restriction work? A study conducted by Dr. Jeff Volek and researchers at the University of Connecticut showed that a diet low in carbohydrates helped more than 70 percent of the men in the study lose more weight and fat than the group on a low-fat diet, despite the fact they ate more calories. The study also showed that a low-carb diet was more effective at removing fat from the body's midsection, important because excess abdominal fat contributes to a higher risk for heart disease.

In another study conducted by Donald Layman and his colleagues at the University of Illinois at Urbana-Champaign, overweight women who ate a higher-protein/lower-carbohydrate diet (40 percent carbs/30 percent protein/30 percent fat) lost less muscle mass than the women who ate according to the U.S. Department of Agriculture (USDA) Food Guide Pyramid (55 percent carbohydrates/15 percent protein/30 percent fat). Layman concluded, "The protein diet was twice as effective. Women eating the lower-protein diet were less capable of burning calories at the end of the study as when they started it. We believe this is the effect of more protein, particularly the increased amount of leucine (an essential amino acid found in protein) in the diet."

Atkins Unless you've been on a pop culture diet for the last few years, you probably know the guy most responsible for the recent low-carb diet craze is Dr. Robert Atkins. Atkins, a cardiologist, first came to national attention back in 1972 when he wrote *Dr. Atkins' Diet Revolution,* which promoted the benefits of a controlled carbohydrate diet. The controversial book was a best-seller, but the low-carb diet didn't really sweep the United States until 2001, when Americans were ready to swap their low-fat breads and pastas for plates of bacon and eggs.

The Atkins plan is one of the more controversial diet plans out there. Much of what Atkins advised in his book contradicted what the rest of the medical and science community said about obesity, heart disease, and other diet-related health conditions. Atkins claimed fat wasn't making people fat, but their reliance on carbohydrates was to blame. The American diet was too dependent on processed and refined foods such as breads, sugar, pasta, and starchy vegetables. This dependence, he believed, was what was behind the rising epidemic of heart attacks, strokes, diabetes, obesity, and other health problems plaguing Americans. His research showed that when dieters replaced typical diet-friendly foods such as pastas and breads with nutrient-dense foods such as meat, fish, poultry, eggs, and vegetables, the pounds dropped off and health conditions such as hypertension and diabetes improved.

His nutritional advice struck a chord with dieters, who were ravenously hungry after years of nibbling on bags of baby carrots with low-fat dip. Not only could you eat typically diet-verboten foods on Atkins—steaks, hamburgers, eggs fried in butter, and cheese—but you didn't have to count calories or weigh portions. You could eat till you were full. Let's face it: fat tastes good, and it's filling. Unlike a box of cookies or a bag of carrots, there are only so many eggs you can eat in one sitting.

The Atkins diet is a four-step process to weight loss. During the first period, called *induction,* the dieter is limited to 20 grams of carbohydrates per day for a minimum of 2 weeks, mostly in the form of salad greens. Contrast that with another diet that recommends 40 percent of daily calorie intake comes from carbohydrates. On a 1,500-calorie-diet plan, you'd be eating 150 grams of carbohydrates. On Atkins, this means no breads, pastas, grains, starchy vegetables, fruits, or sweets, but on the other hand, you're allowed to eat liberal amounts of permitted foods, such as meat, shellfish, cheese, and butter. With so few carbohydrates to burn for fuel, the body turns to burning fat for energy, which puts the dieter into a state of *ketosis.*

PsychSpeak

Ketosis is a condition during which the bloodstream has abnormally high levels of ketones, or what fat is transformed into when it's used as fuel. Dieters who follow Atkins want to achieve ketosis, which can be determined through a urine test.

During these 2 weeks of induction, many dieters experience immediate weight loss, anywhere from a few pounds to 15 pounds or more. This can give them the psychological motivation to stick with the diet. Moreover, because they're eating a diet rich in protein and fat, they tend to feel more full and satisfied.

The second phase, called *ongoing weight loss* (or OWL in Atkins-speak), gradually adds more carbs to the diet—an increase of 5 grams per week. Weight comes off more slowly during this time.

When you're 10 pounds away from your target weight goal, you enter the third phase of Atkins, called *premaintenance*. Now you increase your daily carb count by 10 grams each week. You also start to add fruits back into your diet.

When you've hit your target weight, that's when you enter the fourth phase, *lifetime maintenance*. You know how many carbs you can eat each day without gaining, and you can eat banned foods in moderation (the exception being sugar).

Does Atkins work? You'll certainly find a lot of anecdotal evidence that it does. Ask anyone who has lost 30, 40, 50 pounds or more on the diet, and you're likely to spend as many minutes listening to them sing the praises of a high-fat, low-carb diet: they can eat foods that keep them from feeling gnawingly hungry and still lose weight, the pounds come off fast, and it's easy to do if you're not into fruits and veggies.

The research on Atkins, however, isn't as glowing. A 2003 study published by the *New England Journal of Medicine* showed that although low-carb/high-fat dieters lost more weight than low-fat dieters in the first 6 months of dieting, at the end of the next 6 months, both diets ended up in a statistical dead heat for effectiveness. In a second study, published in 2004 in the *Annals of Internal Medicine,* results showed low-carb dieters kept off the weight they lost the first 6 months, but the low-fat dieters caught up to them by continuing to lose weight over the second 6 months. Not enough long-term studies have been done on Atkins to answer questions as to whether weight loss is sustainable and whether it's safe. Both studies showed that the low-carb/high-fat Atkins diet had the same effect on "bad" LDL cholesterol levels as the low-fat diets and did better on lowering other blood fats than the low-fat diets, including triglycerides. The American Heart Association, which does not prescribe a diet, merely eating guidelines, still recommends that for heart health, a diet low in unsaturated fats is best.

People who follow Atkins often have some short-term problems with the diet. Because it's low in fiber many dieters suffer with constipation. Therefore, it's vitally important to drink a lot of water with this diet. Another side effect is halitosis; high-protein diets tend to give dieters very nasty breath.

The South Beach Diet When President Bill Clinton revealed his new slim self in 2004, everyone wanted to know how this man, known for his love of fast-food burgers and fried foods, took off the weight. The credit went to *The South Beach Diet,* which came fast on the heels of the revised Atkins diet in 2003.

Written by Miami Beach, Florida, cardiologist Arthur Agatston, the South Beach plan is similar to Atkins' in that it promotes a low-carb lifestyle. Agatston developed the diet when he noticed his heart patients weren't responding to low-fat diets typically recommended by cardiologists to patients suffering from heart and other vascular problems. He began to study insulin resistance and how it could be overcome through diet. This led to his development of the South Beach plan.

The South Beach Diet claims it's not a low-carb plan; it insists it teaches dieters how to choose "good carbs" and "good fats." Nevertheless, during the first phase of the diet, you're not allowed to eat bread, rice, potatoes, pasta, baked goods, or fruit to eliminate cravings. Sound familiar? The difference between it and Atkins is that South Beach does not promote a diet of saturated fats. Dieters are encouraged to eat lean meats, chicken, turkey, and shellfish— no bacon, cream, and pork rinds on *this* eating plan.

Like many women, Jean T., 57, didn't have to worry about her weight until she hit middle age. "I was a tiny girl through my teens and 20s," she says, "but then I had some health problems at the end of my 30s that caused me to gain weight." When she quit a job she loved in Washington and began to spend more time at home in the suburbs, she noticed she continued to gain. "I was bored and unhappy," she says. "I was miserable. Life is tough when you're unhappy with yourself." She tried diets, but nothing really seemed to stick. And carrying a lot of weight wasn't easy on her frame. "I'm not quite 5'2". When I noticed that a size 14 was starting to feel tight, I thought, *I've got to do something.*"

The turning point came when Jean and her husband moved south. "I love the Florida lifestyle," she says, "and I love the clothing. I wanted to have that nice Florida look." She was also an avid golfer and noticed that her new friends were fit and trim, so for her, "It was incentive to not be the fat one in the group." Around the time of the realization, Jean read *The South Beach Diet*. Although the plan made sense to her, she modified it for her own tastes and preferences. For example, she loves fruit, and she wasn't willing to give it up, even for the first 2 weeks when fruit is banned. She also enjoyed a glass or two of wine in the evenings. And having done other diet programs such as Weight Watchers in the past, she pulled in weight-loss strategies that worked for her, such as filling up on healthy, low-cal soups to eliminate hunger pains.

Jean lost 40 pounds and kept it off. She also works out three times a week at her local gym to give herself muscle definition and takes 2-mile early morning walks around the golf course. And as a nice bonus, in the past year and a half her golf game has improved. "I've got a high energy level, and I'm constantly on the move," she says. "I'm up at 6:30 A.M., and I don't sit down again till 6:00 P.M."

In the second phase of South Beach, whole-grain breads, pastas, and fruits are reintroduced to the diet. The third phase of the plan shows dieters how to maintain the weight for a lifetime.

Like Atkins, South Beach provides plenty of anecdotal evidence that the plan works. One of the criticisms researchers have with the book is that although it's filled with success stories, there's little in the way of hard research to back up its claims. In a 2003 article in the respected *Harvard Health Letter,* the diet was criticized for its lack of proof and dubious claims. It noted that Dr. Agatston tested the diet on 40 overweight volunteers and presented his findings at the American College of Cardiology, but they pointed out it was too small of a study to use as proof that the diet works. It summed up its review of the diet by saying, "The South Beach Diet is not outlandish, and it may work for some. But like every other diet book that has come along, it makes long-term weight loss seem easier than it is."

The Zone Diet Developed by Barry Sears, Ph.D., as a "drug" to fight heart disease and diabetes, the Zone Diet also promises weight loss and increased energy. It's not so much a low-carb diet, but a diet in which carbohydrates, proteins, and fats are consumed in the "right ratio." By eating in the correct ratio, Sears claims hormones that control weight can be manipulated. It works on the theory that excess insulin, which helps control blood sugar levels, makes you fat. By regulating blood sugar, the body burns fat more efficiently, and you lose weight.

Acceptable foods on this diet include poultry, fish, veal, low-fat dairy products, oatmeal, egg whites, and some fruits and vegetables. The Zone limits most grains and grain products and starchy fruits and vegetables. Every meal should contain 40 percent carbohydrates, 30 percent protein, and 30 percent fat. To help with figuring out this ratio, the diet has specified "zone blocks"—a set amount of food that can be consumed with each meal, depending on your size. The bigger you are, the more blocks you eat. The tough part of this diet is figuring out what makes a block—which is why the marketers behind the Zone Diet have created prepackaged foods to make it easier for dieters.

The Zone Diet can be a lot of work, trying to figure out what food makes a block. On the plus side, it has fewer "no-nos" than the South Beach or Atkins food plans. But it can be complicated to figure out—and expensive if you decide to purchase Zone-friendly prepackaged meals and snacks. Critics point out that it works because it's low in calories—and reducing calories makes you lose weight, not eating foods in the "correct" combination.

Fat Restriction

Remember back in the 1990s when packaged foods proclaimed "0 fat grams" or "fat-free"? As Americans turned to eating more fat-free and low-fat foods, obesity levels continued to rise. In fact, obesity rates doubled in the 1990s!

The problem is that many dieters turned to fat-free and low-fat packaged foods, thinking they could eat as much as they wanted and still lose weight. To compensate for the fat-reduction, food manufacturers added more sugar to their products. While the foods were often low-fat, they were also high-calorie. And that goes back to one of the dieting truths: you will gain weight when you take in more calories than your body can burn off.

Most dietary experts recommend that no matter what you weigh, you should watch your fat intake. The USDA recommends a diet low in fats, especially saturated fats. You should get less than 30 percent of your daily calories from fat. If you're trying to lose weight, that percentage should be lower.

To figure out how many fat calories to consume each day, follow these guidelines: if your calorie target is 1,800 calories per day, you should aim to consume no more than 540 fat calories per day. If you're counting fat grams, 540 calories translates into 60 grams of fat (60 grams of fat × 9 calories per gram = 540 calories).

I'm confused. I've always thought fat was bad for you, but I've been hearing a lot about "good fats" and "bad fats." Isn't fat just fat?

No, it isn't. Dietary fat comes in four different types:

- *Monounsaturated fats* are the fats you find in olive and canola oils. These fats can help you reduce LDL cholesterol and maintain your HDL cholesterol, the good cholesterol.

- *Polyunsaturated fats* are in vegetable oils, nuts, and some fish. These fats can reduce blood cholesterol as well.

- *Saturated fats* are found in meat, milk, and dairy products, as well as a great number of processed foods. Saturated fats raise blood cholesterol, so they should be limited.

- *Trans fatty acids* (or *trans fats*) are man-made fats found in partially hydrogenated vegetable oils, which are used to make margarine and shortening and are included in many processed, packaged foods. These fats raise cholesterol levels. Studies have noted that the increased consumption of trans fats has led to increased rates of heart disease.

Even if the fats being consumed are "good fats," no more than 30 percent of your daily calories should come from them because ingesting a higher percentage of dietary fat is linked with weight gain and the development of health conditions such as heart disease, breast cancer, and type 2 diabetes. Limit the consumption of saturated fats by choosing lean meats and poultry and low-fat dairy products. Avoid trans fats at all costs due to their dismal effects on health.

Your goal shouldn't be to eliminate every gram of fat from your diet. An extreme low-fat diet, like any other extreme diet, won't help you lose weight faster, nor will it keep you healthier. Your body needs dietary fat to rev up weight loss. Fat gives you energy. It keeps your skin smooth, your hair glossy, and your joints lubricated. The right kinds of dietary fats deliver *essential fatty acids (EFAs)* necessary for metabolic function. Fats help you process fat-soluble vitamins such as A, D, E, and K.

PsychSpeak

Your body requires **essential fatty acids (EFAs)** in your diet because these fatty acids cannot be synthesized by your body; your body must obtain EFAs from food. EFAs assist with everything from basic metabolic functions to possibly preventing chronic disease. Omega-3s and omega-6s are EFAs that can be found in vegetable oils, nuts, fish, seeds, and some leafy vegetables.

Dean Ornish If Dr. Atkins's plan is at one end of the spectrum (high-fat/ low-carb), then Dr. Dean Ornish's plan is on the other side (low-fat/high-carbs). Ornish gets a tremendous amount of respect in the medical community for proving that heart disease can be stopped—even reversed— through diet rather than through surgery and/or drugs.

Like Atkins and Agatston, Ornish noted that the typical low-fat/high-carb diet recommended to heart patients wasn't effective. Rather than veer away from the low-fat path as the two other doctors had done, Ornish took low-fat dieting a step further. In his book, *Dr. Dean Ornish's Plan for Reversing Heart Disease,* Dr. Ornish claims that the recommended diet didn't go far enough to make noticeable changes in heart disease patients. A diet of 30 percent fat still supplies too much saturated fat and cholesterol; thus, he recommended patients eat only fruits, vegetables, whole grains, and beans, with a minimal amount of nonfat dairy and egg whites. That's right: no animal fats, no oils, no sugar.

In the past few years, the Ornish plan has not only become a plan for reversing heart disease, but also a weight control plan. As a result, there are two versions: a restrictive one for heart disease patients, and a preventative plan that's far less restrictive. Both plans also include recommendations for stress relief/ meditation, smoking cessation, and exercise. The plan has been so effective at treating heart disease that some insurance companies actually cover the formal 3- to 12-month Ornish program.

Now for the bad news: the Ornish plan is a tough diet to stick to. You have to be really motivated to change your diet so radically, which is why it's probably easier to adopt if you have no other choice but surgery. Moreover, research shows that an ultra-low-fat diet reduces not only bad cholesterol (LDL) but also the good cholesterol (HDL), and in some dieters, it can increase triglycerides. Dieters without heart problems may want to increase the level of "good" dietary fats to offset these drawbacks.

Pritikin Similar to the Ornish plan, the Pritikin plan was developed by a scientist and engineer—Nathan Pritikin—who was looking for a diet-based solution to his own heart problems. The advice doctors were giving to heart patients in the 1950s was to "take it easy." Instead, Pritikin began investigating ways better nutrition and exercise could reverse heart disease and other chronic illnesses. His research showed that people who had cholesterol levels lower than 160 tended not to suffer from heart disease. His own cholesterol was 280, but when he changed his diet—eliminating foods high in saturated fats, for example—his cholesterol dropped to 120 and his doctors pronounced him free of heart disease. In the late 1970s, the medical community took notice of Pritikin's work. In 1975, he founded the Pritikin Longevity Center, a health resort and longevity center for the general public. He also wrote books about his program, many of which soared up the best-seller lists.

The Pritikin Program is comprised of a diet of fruits, vegetables, whole grains, fish, and limited amounts of lean meat. It also advises exercise. By following the plan, dieters can expect to lose weight; lower total cholesterol and "bad" LDL cholesterol; manage insulin levels with diabetes; reduce blood pressure; eliminate the need for heart surgery; and reduce the risk of conditions such as heart disease, obesity, diabetes, and certain cancers.

Hundreds of studies have proven that the Pritikin plan is highly effective at not only helping people lose weight, but also at reducing or eliminating chronic health conditions such as heart disease, type 2 diabetes, and more. Although it doesn't specifically recommend the Pritikin plan, in 2004 the World Health Organization (WHO) developed a Global Strategy on Diet, Physical Activity, and Health, which recommends a diet that limits fats; increases consumption of fruits, vegetables, legumes, whole grains, and nuts; and limits sugars and sodium intake, much like the Pritikin plan does.

But like the Ornish plan, the Pritikin Program can be tough for a lot of dieters to follow over time because of its extreme low-fat regimen. Low-fat food tends to feel less filling, so dieters often feel hungrier. This may be why the plan has been modified to focus on foods that have few calories per pound, so dieters can fill up without the fat.

> *Example:* 100 grams of a Krispy Kreme traditional cake donut contains 386 calories. But 100 grams of a raw apple contains only 52 calories. Guess which food you can eat more of.

Nutritionists and doctors also point out that a diet in which less than 10 percent of the calories come from fat can be difficult to maintain—food preparation takes a lot of extra planning, and let's face it, Americans like to eat out. Being that vigilant over fat content can take an enormous amount of dedication.

Sugar Restriction

There's no denying human beings have sweet tooths. Sugar consumption continues to rise each year, not only in the United States but around the world. The Food and Agriculture Organization of the United Nations forecasts that sugar consumption in 2004/2005 will exceed global sugar production for the second year in a row. The average American eats 20 teaspoons of sugar a day—double what the USDA advises for people following a 2,000-calorie-a-day diet.

In response, diets advising the restriction of sugar intake have grown in popularity. These plans advise cutting out all refined sugar—such as white sugar, corn syrup, and honey—from the diet and staying away from other foods high on the *glycemic index*—such as white flour. Such approaches advocate a diet rich in veggies, fruits, and whole grains, as long as they're low on the glycemic index. It's also okay to eat lean meats, fish, and dairy products.

PsychSpeak

Glycemic index (or **GI**) is a measure of a food's ability to raise blood sugar levels. Foods low on the index raise blood sugars minimally, whereas foods high on the index raise blood sugars. A steady diet of high-glycemic foods can promote obesity and diabetes.

The theory behind a sugar-restriction diet is that when you ingest sugar, it creates excess insulin in your body, which prevents you from losing weight even if you exercise. Proponents of sugar restriction claim that high levels of sugar intake are not only responsible for our country's increasing obesity problem, but are also to blame for other health conditions plaguing Americans, including diabetes, heart disease, and cancer.

Nutrition experts have a few concerns about sugar restriction diets. First, although most doctors and nutritionists agree that cutting back on sugar is a great step to losing weight, there's no evidence that sugar is the cause of excessive weight. Moreover, there's no evidence sugar is responsible for the host of ills anti-sugar advocates blame on it. As the *Harvard Health Letter* pointed out in a 2005 review of popular diets, refined sugars aren't toxic; they just add unnecessary calories. Another challenge is the difficulty in avoiding a whole category of food, especially for a lifetime—no more white bread, no more potatoes, no more corn. It's also a diet that requires an enormous amount of commitment and dedication: every package of food must be scrutinized for ingredients such as fructose, corn syrup, honey, or other sweeteners.

Moreover, there's some controversy among experts over the value of the glycemic index. Case in point: carrots. Carrots, according to sugar-restriction proponents, are high on the glycemic index and, thus, should be avoided. The diet's opponents point out that carrots are also loaded with antioxidants that protect against cardiovascular disease and cancer. They're also a good source of vitamin C, dietary fiber, and potassium. In their view, telling Americans not to eat carrots is just another way to limit people from eating healthy complex carbohydrates.

What You Can Do

Cut calories? Cut carbs? Cut fats? A tremendous amount of controversy exists about what type of restriction diet works best for dieters, so the decision is up to you. Restriction diets do work; the challenge is figuring out which restriction diet will work for you and will help keep the weight off forever.

☐ Before going on any diet, talk it over with a health-care professional first.

☐ Keep this in mind: most diets work for some people some of the time. If you're a person who can't give up cheese and meats, a low-carb diet is probably a plan you're more likely to stick to. Whatever plan you choose, keep its draw-backs in mind so you can make adjustments as necessary.

☐ Pay attention to the healthy eating patterns you have today. Look for a restriction plan that supports the healthy eating trends you enjoy—not the ones you wish you had.

☐ Fully research restriction plans that look attractive to you. Read the books. Surf the Net. Talk to friends and family. Anecdotal advice does have its place in decision-making.

☐ Think baby steps. There's no law that says you have to embrace a formal diet plan fully. If you notice there's too much sugar in your diet, work to cut it out slowly rather than going whole-hog on the plan. Use only the elements of the plan that make sense for you. You can also pull good advice from one plan (limiting simple carbs such as sugars and white flour) and combine it with another plan's good advice (eating more lean sources of protein).

Lifestyle Diets

The word *diet* encompasses the sum of the food we consume every day. For many of you reading this book, however, the word has another meaning. It means giving up a few of your favorite foods, or cutting back on food portions. Diet, for you, stands for deprivation and hard work.

For some people, the two meanings of the word meet at a crossroads. The food they consume every day is a big part of the way they live their lives. Their food choices are tied up in their beliefs—about religion, culture, economics, health, recreation, and/or ethics. A person who is impassioned about corporate farming practices or who has strong opinions about the humane treatment of animals, for example, usually makes dietary choices based on those beliefs. These beliefs drive the way you live your life, and these beliefs, therefore, have to be accommodated when weight loss must be achieved.

It is possible to lose weight safely and effectively on a diet that upholds a person's beliefs and lifestyle choices. In fact, sometimes it's easier to accommodate weight loss with these diets. For example, if you eat a vegetarian diet, cutting out excess animal fat from your diet is a nonissue. If you're already happy with the way you live your life and most of the foods you eat, your weight-loss plan may require only minor shifts rather than seismic changes.

The Pros and Cons of Lifestyle Diets

When your personal beliefs dictate how you eat, you already have something of a food plan in place, which may make dieting easier for you than for someone who doesn't have certain rules or guidelines about food in place. You already know what you will or won't eat, which can make dieting and, thus, losing weight, easier.

On the other hand, you may be more limited in your weight-loss choices. You may have certain food restrictions. If you're a vegetarian and decide you want to cut carbs and boost protein,

you're not alone

I was raised as a vegetarian in a commune, where I picked up very healthy attitudes about food and physical activity—dance and movement were really important. As a child and teen, I was thin. Then I moved overseas and lived in urban areas in places such as Italy, Ireland, and India, where I didn't need a car—I was always a pedestrian. And I kept up the vegetarian diet.

When I was in India, I developed a gastrointestinal disease, which kept me from eating many kinds of vegetables, beans, and lentils, so that's when

I started eating meat. When I came back to the United States, I moved to a place where it was necessary to have a car, so I didn't move as much. And unfortunately, that's when I started eating fried foods. At this point, I was around 150 or 160 pounds and thought I was 'fat.' Eventually I maxed out at 284 pounds.

In March 2004, I decided to do something about my weight and my health. My blood pressure was high, and I started thinking about stuff such as *Is this cupcake worth having a heart attack at*

50? My thinking was in terms of questions, rather than thinking 'size 5' or 'size 7.' My initial goal was to lose 10 percent of my weight (29 pounds). After I did that, I noticed a difference. I slept better, I had more energy, and I felt mentally alert. I loved feeling strong.

I designed my own plan, doing a lot of research on my own, and combining the best of a number of plans. I ate 5 or 6 meals a day, focusing on a low-calorie, low-fat, and low-sodium diet. I ate minimal amounts of refined sugar and high-

that's going to take some work, especially if you don't eat eggs or dairy. And although accepting a diet based on beliefs may be easier, it certainly isn't easy. Dieting doesn't have to be misery, but it's rarely easy. As you'll read later in this chapter, people who believe in Calorie Restriction, or CR, to lengthen their lives often obsess about food.

Vegetarianism

The practice of vegetarianism has a long, distinguished history although the term *vegetarian* didn't come about until 1847, when the Vegetarian Society of the United Kingdom was established.

glycemic foods, while eating lots of fiber and getting 40 percent of my calories from protein. My exercise regimen was tough: I did intensity intervals with my cardiovascular exercise, which I did 3 to 5 times per week. And I developed some good habits such as 'batch cooking' so I could portion out my meals and have them ready when I needed them. I also tracked my food with a software program called *Diet Power*.

By the time December 2004 rolled around, I'd lost 80 pounds in 9 months. Then I was diagnosed with Hodgkin's disease and had to begin a regimen of chemotherapy. Having lost all that weight and being healthy at that moment was a blessing. My doctor actually said, "Thank God you've lost weight," because it meant I could better weather the chemo treatments. And because I learned how to control my eating and exercise, it helped me cope with the diagnosis. I had learned through controlling my weight that a day is just a whole pile of moments and that I can see something through to the other side. I just have to do one thing at a time.

I haven't been able to stick to my eating and exercise plan since the diagnosis, and I miss it. The chemotherapy has left me extremely fatigued, and I'm taking steroids that have caused some weight gain. But I know, without a doubt, when my treatments end, I'm going right back to my eating plan. I can't wait. I love the routine, I love the healthy attitude I developed, and I love that I have taken active leadership in my health. —*Sarah H., 41, Baltimore, Maryland*

Ancient Hindu teachings prohibited the eating of flesh, and a number of Greek philosophers and thinkers, including Plato and Socrates, eschewed meat. Voltaire, Alexander Pope, George Bernard Shaw, and John Wesley (who founded Methodism) were all vegetarians. Today it's not uncommon to hear about sports figures or celebrities having "gone veg."

According to the *Journal of the American Dietetic Association*, 2.5 percent of Americans follow a vegetarian diet; that is, a diet that contains no meat, fish, or fowl. Many people go veggie for health reasons, citing evidence a plant-based diet is lower in saturated fats and cholesterol and contains beneficial levels of fiber, antioxidants, phytochemicals, and other substances. Other vegetarians choose the lifestyle because they are strong believers in animal welfare. Some vegetarians don't eat meat because of their religious beliefs, and others don't eat meat because of ethical concerns with farming and world hunger. Still others just don't like the taste of meat and/or animal products. And usually there's some crossover within these groups.

There are three types of vegetarian eating patterns:

- *Lacto-ovo vegetarians* eat grains, vegetables, fruits, legumes, seeds, nuts, dairy, and eggs, but exclude meat, fish, and fowl from their diets.
- *Lacto vegetarians* eat grains, vegetables, fruits, legumes, seeds, nuts, and dairy, but exclude eggs, meat, fish, and fowl from their diets.
- *Vegans* eat grains, vegetables, fruits, legumes, seeds, and nuts. They exclude eggs, dairy, meat, fish, fowl, and other animal products from their diets and lifestyles.

Some recognize a fourth type of vegetarian, which we'll call the *semi-vegetarian*. These self-described "vegetarians" occasionally eat meat, fish, and fowl, but mostly eat a plant-based diet.

It's far easier to be a vegetarian today than it was 30 years ago. The National Restaurant Association reports that 8 out of 10 restaurants in the United States offer vegetarian entrées. Grocery store shelves are stocked with a variety of flavorful vegetarian products, including soy and rice milks, yogurts, meat substitutes, seasoned tofu, and easy-to-cook grains. An ever greater variety of fruits and vegetables is also offered, thanks to developments in air freighting. Vegetarianism has become so mainstream that it's not uncommon to find vegetarian cookbooks on the shelves of meat-eating home cooks. An interest in foods and cooking from different cultures has also shown us that veggie-based meals can be nutritious, delicious, and filling.

With everyone from the American Cancer Society, the American Heart Association, and the National Institutes of Health urging Americans to eat more grains and vegetables, a vegetarian diet has a number of advantages for dieters. In past years, there was some concern that vegetarians had a hard time getting complete proteins in their diet. That challenge seems to have been solved with the availability of a greater variety of vegetable-based complete proteins. Our vegetarian parents had to get creative with the bland blocks of tofu available at their local health-food stores. However, we, their vegetarian sons and daughters, can walk into almost any supermarket and find everything from barbecue-flavored soy "meat," tofu hot dogs—even soy-based ice cream and yogurt! Moreover, many foods—even those marketed to nonvegetarians—are fortified with those additional nutrients, vitamins, and minerals vegetarians commonly need. For example, there is orange juice fortified with calcium, vitamins E and D—even extra vitamin C. Sometimes buying a simple carton of orange juice isn't so simple!

If you're already eating a vegetarian diet and you want to lose weight, it can be done. Vegetarian dieters need to pay special attention to their diet, however, says Lisa Dorfman, M.S., R.D., L.M.H.C, author of *The Vegetarian Sports Nutrition Guide*. First, there's portion size. "Vegetarian dieters may assume because they're not eating meat, they can eat as much as they want because 'they need it,'" she says. Not so. "They still need to watch those calories, so monitoring portion size is going to be key."

WEB TALK: Check out the vegetarian food pyramid and eating guidelines at:
www.eatright.org/Public/NutritionInformation/92_17086.cfm

On top of that, dieting vegetarians have to make smarter food choices. "You need to get more out of what you're eating," says Dorfman, "so look for nutrient-dense foods. You want foods that have color: the deep reds and browns of whole grains, the rich yellows of squash and peppers." She also urges vegetarians to take advantage of fortification. When you ensure every mouthful of food is packed with nutrients—not just calories—you can better meet weight-loss goals.

What if you're thinking of both losing weight and going vegetarian? Can it be done? It can, but it'll be a challenge. Dieting is already hard enough without adding an extra layer of change to the diet, says Dorfman. If you're gung-ho on the idea, here's what she recommends:

- Tune up the eating habits you have today. If you're hitting the fast-food counters at lunchtime and think you'll have no trouble heading for the salad bar instead, think again. Instead, wean yourself off fast foods by making better lunchtime choices—such as packing your own lunch or switching to a restaurant that offers healthier food choices.

- Start eating a wider variety of plant-based foods. "Vegetarianism calls for open-mindedness," says Dorfman. "You just can't be eating apples and lettuce, or switch to eating breads and pastas—you have to eat beans and explore new grains."

- Make a gradual transition to vegetarianism. Instead of going cold turkey on meat, start by eating 1 or 2 vegetarian meals per week. When you're comfortable with that, add a third meal, and so on.

Paleolithic Diet

We've seen a lot of changes in the past 30,000 years, but most scientists will agree that the genes in our bodies today differ little from the genes of our ancient ancestors. What has changed? The foods we eat. Fifty-five percent of the foods we eat today simply weren't available to our ancient forefathers and foremothers. Wheat, potatoes, corn, sugar, and milk—some of these were not available until 10,000 years ago, when our ancestors finally figured out how to cultivate land and domesticate animals. And therein, many experts say, is where our dietary problems started.

A small yet vocal band of researchers and evolutionary nutritionists claim the conditions that run rampant in our society—such as obesity, heart disease, diabetes, auto-immune disorders, cancer, and even depression—were virtually unheard of in the days when our ancestors hunted and gathered their food. Those early men and women ate a diet high in protein, complemented by moderate amounts of complex carbohydrates from fruits and veggies. What's more, the meat came from animals of the wild—far leaner, much chewier, and with a vastly healthier makeup of fats. Basically, they ate the USDA food pyramid turned upside down. The average caveman lived for only 20 years, but that was due more to a harsh life than poor diet. Research shows these people were quite healthy. In parts of the world even today, hunter/gatherer societies are free of modern-day illnesses. Interestingly, their diets are very similar to those eaten 30,000 years ago.

WEB TALK: Learn more about the origins and evolution of human diet at:

www.cast.uark.edu/local/icaes/index.html

The solution, these researchers say, is to eat the same foods our fitter, healthier ancestors ate. Known in popular literature as the Paleo Diet, the Caveman Diet, and the Paleothin Diet, a Paleolithic diet consists of eating only meats (preferably grass-fed), fish, eggs, fruits, vegetables, berries, and nuts. It banishes grains, beans, rice, potatoes, dairy products, and sugar from the dinner plate.

Two researchers from Purdue University and Colorado State University published research in the *European Journal of Clinical Nutrition* about the chemical analysis of meats eaten 10,000 years ago. They looked at wild game from the Rockies, such as venison, elk, and antelope, and compared them to meats taken from grain-fed and grass-fed beef. The wild game and grass-fed beef contained higher amounts of omega-6 and omega-3 fatty acids in a ratio that would lower cholesterol and reduce the risk of chronic disease, while the grain-fed beef contained more saturated fats.

And therein lies the difficulty of adopting a Paleolithic diet. It's certainly easier to procure grass-fed meat today than it was 10 years ago. Many supermarkets sell grass-fed bison meat (more commonly known as buffalo), which is lower in saturated fat than beef, in their specialty meats departments. However, if you have a hankering for beef, the steaks, roasts, and ground meats you'll find there and at your local butcher will probably be from grain-fed animals whose meats don't have the healthy ratio of essential fatty acids. It also means eliminating all grains, potatoes, beans, and sugar except that found in fruit. Adopting a true Paleolithic diet takes time, commitment, and most likely, some extra money.

The jury is out on the health benefits of a Paleolithic diet. Certainly, a diet rich in whole, unprocessed foods gets a thumbs-up from doctors and nutritionists. Eliminating empty carbs such as those found in white bread, pasta, and sweets will go far in helping you reach your weight-loss and health goals. However, no scientific evidence exists that says the carbohydrates found in whole grains and beans cause the medical illnesses and health conditions that Paleolithic proponents say they do. In fact, most nutritionists urge dieters to include more whole grains and beans in their diets for their vitamins, minerals, and fiber.

WEB TALK: Read more about paleolithic diets at: www.paleodiet.com

The "Calorie Restriction" Movement

Imagine living 120 years—or beyond—in good health. Science fiction or reality?

Reality, according to some scientists who've studied how calorie restriction, or CR, has increased the lifespan of a variety of animals, including protozoa, guppies, rats, mice, and dogs. Research shows that when calorie intake is cut 25 to 30 percent in these animals while maintaining adequate nutrition, their lifespan increases anywhere from 10 to 40 percent due to biochemical changes that delay aging. Moreover, these calorie-restricted animals enjoy good health. Laboratory studies have shown that caloric restriction in animals inhibits the growth of tumors, reduces the risk of diabetes and cardiovascular disease, and improves memory, especially later in life.

WEB TALK: Learn more about CR at: www.calorierestriction.org/

Several theories exist as to why CR extends life. First, extreme calorie restriction slows metabolism, a built-in evolutionary response that helps conserve energy when food isn't available. Metabolism, which is the burning of glucose to create energy, is what gives us our "get up and go"; metabolism also produces *free radicals,* unstable atoms and molecules that can damage and destroy healthy cells. Free radicals occur naturally, and our bodies have systems in place to cope with them, but over time, damage from free radicals contributes to aging and disease. CR also lowers the core body temperature of primates, creating an inhospitable environment for disease. Some evidence also exists that cells simply work better on less energy, and that CR affects gene expression in test animals, preventing or slowing expression of genes later in life. How does this research impact humans? Say you're genetically programmed to develop Alzheimer's disease during your lifetime. Followers of CR would tell you that by cutting calorie intake, you'd delay—or even halt—the timer in your genes that triggers this disease.

PsychSpeak

A **free radical** is an atom or molecule that has been rendered unstable or highly reactive because of its unpaired electron. These atoms or molecules grab electrons from molecules in healthy cells, thus damaging the cell. Free radicals are linked to aging, heart disease, and cancer.

Researchers at the National Institute on Aging and the University of Wisconsin are conducting long-term studies on how CR impacts rhesus monkeys, whose DNA is similar to humans'. The studies aren't complete, but the early results look promising. In the NIA study, which began in 1987, two control monkeys are dying for every one CR monkey. And in the University of Wisconsin study, the CR monkeys are leaner and more insulin-sensitive than the control monkeys.

Long life and great health. What's not to love? Eager to use themselves as guinea pigs, a number of people have started practicing CR themselves by consuming anywhere from 1,200 to 1,600 calories a day on a permanent basis, depending on their sex and size. Because CR reduces the percentage of calories of a healthy, balanced diet—it's not simply cutting portion sizes or eating less—the pounds drop away slowly, due to the slowing of metabolism. The benefits not only include a low BMI, lowered cholesterol, and better blood sugar levels, but some CR advocates claim they feel more calm, have better memories, and think more clearly on fewer calories.

Now the downside: we all know how tough it can be to eat less. Following a CR diet takes an enormous amount of willpower and discipline, which makes it a tough lifestyle diet to adopt. CR followers report they often obsess about food, or lack of it, especially as they begin the diet. There are also other side effects, such as lowered body temperature, which leaves dieters feeling cold all the time and lowers libido. Women dieters may experience missed periods, infertility, and bone loss.

Although the research on primates looks promising, no long-term CR studies have been performed on humans.

GET PSYCHED

"[Calorie restriction] takes a lot of self-discipline that not many people in our society have. And that's unfortunate because I think it has a lot of health benefits and a lot of psychological benefits. I'm in it for the adventure. I enjoy doing something different from everyone else." –Dean Pomerleau, CR follower, in Psychology Today, May/June 2004

Raw Foods

Isn't "raw foodist" just another term for a vegetarian? Yes and no. A raw foodist is someone who only eats plant-based foods that are uncooked or minimally cooked, unprocessed, and preferably organically grown. Their diets typically consist of fruits, vegetables, sprouts, nuts, seeds, grains, and sea vegetables. Nuts, seeds, and grains are usually soaked in water before they're eaten. Raw foodists believe that uncooked foods provide *enzymes* cooked foods can't. In fact, some raw foodists go so far as to believe cooked foods are toxic.

Some raw foodists only eat fruits; others only eat sprouts; still others drink only juices. People become raw foodists for a variety of reasons. Some are convinced a diet of raw foods is healthier for them, kinder to the environment, and respectful of world food resources. Others go "raw" because they've heard raw foods can cure diseases ranging from auto-immune disorders to cancers.

PsychSpeak

An **enzyme** is a protein or conjugated protein produced by living organisms; it functions as a biochemical catalyst. Enzymes in food assist with digestion and nutrient absorption within the body.

On the plus side, there's no denying a diet rich in fruits and vegetables delivers powerful health benefits. You'll be getting lots of valuable vitamins, minerals, phytochemicals, and dietary fiber. And if you aim to eat all organic foodstuffs, you'll further reduce your contact with pesticides, growth hormones, and irradiation. You're also better off without the saturated fats, cholesterol, and trans fats your friends who eat meat and processed foods get in their diets.

But there are also some minuses. First, an all or mostly all raw-foods diet requires a lot of discipline and commitment. You've got to find the time to sprout seeds and grains. If you live in a cold climate, it can be difficult and expensive during the off-season to consume a variety of fresh fruits and vegetables. Eating out can be a challenge, although you can certainly order salads or try one of the new raw foods establishments sprouting up in major metropolitan areas. Whenever you limit food choices—in this case, any food cooked above 160 degrees Fahrenheit—you run the risk of getting bored with your eating plan. You must be ever curious about experimenting with raw foods.

There's also little evidence that a diet of raw foods is better for you than, say, a vegetarian diet—and in fact it could be bad for your health. The American Dietetic Association points out that the body already produces the necessary enzymes needed to digest and absorb food; there's no biochemical rationale for eating raw foods. It also points out that sprouts are often grown in environments that can promote unhealthy bacteria. Moreover, eating foods that haven't been cooked at proper temperatures can lead to food-borne illness. Couple these cautions with the limits this diet puts on some food groups—proteins, for example—and you may be depleting your body of the valuable nutrients it needs. You may even get too many nutrients, especially if you turn to a juice diet. Fruits, for example, are high in sugars, which you probably don't need a lot of if you're trying to lose weight. If you're juicing them, you're leaving all the fruit's fibers behind, which actually help slow the absorption of fruit sugars.

Cooking actually maximizes the nutritional benefits of many vegetables and some fruits. In research presented to the American Chemical Society in 2000, the bioavailability of iron was improved in 37 of the 48 cooked vegetables studied. For example, the iron bioavailability of broccoli flowerets was quite low when uncooked (6 percent) but it jumped to more than 30 percent when cooked. When you keep in mind that iron deficiency can be a problem for dieters, it makes a strong case for heating—and eating—those veggies.

The Macrobiotic Diet

When many people hear *macrobiotic diet* they often think *anti-cancer*. In the last 20 years, the diet has been credited in books and the media for halting, even reversing, cancer and other life-threatening diseases in people for whom conventional medicine has failed. More recently, the diet has undergone a revival and facelift because of news that super-fit celebrities such as Madonna and Gwyneth Paltrow follow it.

Developed in the 1930s by George Ohsawa, a Japanese philosopher, macrobiotics is founded on ancient Far Eastern teachings. According to followers, a macrobiotic diet promotes balance and harmony in health and diet through the opposing yet complementary forces of yin and yang. When yin and yang forces are out of balance, disease and disharmony result.

Foods in the macrobiotic diet are classified as yin or yang: yin foods are cool; yang foods are hot. Some foods are classified as "too yin" or "too yang," and practitioners of macrobiotics avoid them. In the "too yin" corner you'll find sugar, strong spices, alcohol, and caffeine; over in the yang corner are meat, poultry, eggs, and dairy products. Followers eat a balance of "good yin" foods, such as seasonal—and preferably locally grown—fruits and veggies, sea vegetables, and tofu to balance out "good yang" foods, such as brown rice, whole grains, legumes, miso soup, and minimal amounts of fish and shellfish.

The nutritional composition of a macrobiotic diet is 50 percent whole grains; 25 percent seasonal veggies; 10 percent soy, legumes, and fish for protein; 5 percent sea vegetables; 5 percent soups, especially miso, a soybean paste broth; and 5 percent nuts, seeds, fruits, and drinks. It's low in calories and high in fiber and complex carbohydrates. It's also low in saturated fats;

the fats you ingest on a macrobiotic diet come from heart-healthy essential fatty acids (EFAs).

Some studies show that people who eat a macrobiotic diet have fewer heart problems and avoid certain types of cancers. Unfortunately, there's little to no scientific evidence backing up

WEB TALK: For more information and support on the macrobiotic diet, visit:

www.cybermacro.com/

anecdotal claims that a macrobiotic diet can halt or reverse cancer. The American Cancer Society says some aspects of a macrobiotic diet can benefit cancer patients—whole grains, fruits, and vegetables, for example—but again, they also say there's no reliable data to prove that a macrobiotic diet works better than the diet they recommend to cancer patients. The diet is also seriously deficient in vital nutrients, especially for pregnant and breast-feeding women, infants, and young children. (It is worth pointing out it was widely reported that superslim Gwyneth Paltrow gave up her macrobiotic diet when she was pregnant.) A study conducted in the Netherlands showed that children who followed a macrobiotic diet were seriously deficient in energy, protein, vitamin B_{12}, vitamin D, calcium, and riboflavin. This led to retarded growth, fat and muscle wasting, and slower psychomotor development. Other studies have been conducted in which a macrobiotic diet can lead to rapid weight loss and serious, life-threatening deficiencies in adults.

Athletic Diets

Amateur and professional athletes often follow special diets to support training, athletic events, and weight maintenance. Often, these athletes must lose weight, so their diets must support the energy that's expended during training as well as promote safe weight loss.

Unfortunately, athletes, like dieters, aren't immune to the allure of rapid weight loss. Some of them cut back on energy intake or eliminate one or more food groups from their diets in an effort to "make weight." They'll even cut back on water intake. Because these people subject their bodies to greater stresses than the average dieter, they can become even more vulnerable to nutritional deficiencies and injury.

The American Dietetic Association recommends that athletes pursuing weight loss work with a dietician trained in sports nutrition to help them develop a healthy diet. The weight goal should be one that:

- Can be realistically maintained.
- Allows for improvement in athletic performance.
- Minimizes risk of injury or illness.
- Reduces risk factors for chronic disease.

If you are designing your own athletic performance diet, the ADA offers these suggestions for food intake:

- Decrease energy intake by 10 to 20 percent to begin weight loss without feeling deprived or overly hungry. Use strategies such as substituting lower-fat foods for whole-fat foods and reduce consumption of energy-dense snacks.
- Fat intake should not be decreased below 15 percent of your total energy intake.
- Eat more whole grains and cereals, beans, and legumes.
- Eat 5 or more servings of fruits and vegetables daily.
- Avoid skimping on protein, and keep up adequate calcium intake. Use low-fat dairy products, and choose lean meats, fish, and poultry.

- Drink plenty of water, especially before, during, and after workouts. Dehydration is not the way to lose weight.

- Avoid skipping meals, especially breakfast, and don't let yourself get too hungry. Keep healthful snacks on hand for snacking.

- Keep dietary goals flexible and achievable. According to the ADA, "Athletes should remember that all foods can fit into a healthful lifestyle; however, some foods are chosen less frequently."

- Plan for dietary weaknesses (skipping meals, eating too many energy bars), and figure out strategies to handle them.

- Focus on making lifelong changes to support health and optimal nutrition rather than following a short-term solution.

Some athletic nutrition plans advise the use of herbal and nutritional supplements, meal replacement bars and shakes, and energy drinks. Many of these products, especially the bars and shakes, can help athletes during training and competition. As for the supplements and drinks, proceed with caution. Many of these products have been proven to be ineffective—even dangerous. The FDA doesn't regulate over-the-counter nutritional supplements, so marketers are free to claim what they want about their products. Before you invest a lot of time and money in a product that promises to build lean muscle mass and burn your body fat while you sleep, do some research. Check with a qualified sports nutritionist or your doctor. (See Chapter 6 for more information about dietary and herbal supplements.)

How Healthy Cultures Eat and Stay Slim

When foreigners arrive in America, they're often gobsmacked by the sheer size and abundance of what they see. Everything here is larger than what they're used to in their own countries: not just the cities and land, but our grocery stores, our people, and our portions.

Portion sizes here are much larger than anywhere else in the world. A modest portion of pasta, for example, is usually served as a first course in Italy and is rarely the star attraction of a meal. Courses that follow are also modestly portioned so diners can enjoy a greater variety of foods and flavors without leaving the table feeling "stuffed." Yet here, it's "All You Can Eat Pasta Wednesday." Even if you're not eating buffet style, a main-course pasta dish with its attendant cheeses and meats will often cost you 1,500 calories or more.

For many years, the "French Paradox" has stymied researchers. In general, the French suffer fewer deaths from heart attacks yet have higher cholesterol levels. They certainly don't avoid fat— think creamy bries and braised red meats—but they tend to eat better fats—think olive oil—and watch portion size on the brie and braised meats. They also consume fewer reduced-fat foods than Americans. They drink more red wine, which has led some researchers to explore the link between polyphenols—the compounds that give wine its color and astringent quality—and their cardiovascular benefits. Despite the fact they don't avoid fat and drink more wine, the French are leaner than Americans: only 7.4 percent are considered obese versus 22.3 percent for Americans.

Research points to portion size as a factor. A 2003 study published in the journal *Psychological Science* compared differences in food portion sizes in Paris and Philadelphia. The mean portion size across 11 restaurants in Paris was 277 grams, versus 346 grams in comparable restaurants in Philadelphia—a 25 percent difference. The researchers also compared single-serve foods sold at grocery stores in both cities and found 14 of 17 items studied were larger in the United States. The lead author, Paul Rozin, sums up the findings, "Ironically, although the French eat less than Americans, they seem to eat for a longer period of time, and hence have more food experience. The French can have their cake and eat it as well."

It's worth emphasizing that the French spend more time eating. Americans eat on the run and tend to eat fast. But when you take longer to eat, and savor every morsel, your stomach has time to tell your brain it's full. If you eat fast, your brain doesn't have time to tell your stomach, "Stop!" You end up eating more calories than you need to feel satisfied.

We can learn a lot about nutrition, health, and weight loss from other cultures. Adapting a multicultural approach to food offers American dieters fresh ideas for approaching weight loss.

WEB TALK: Download "healthy eating pyramids" for vegetarian, Asian, Mediterranean, and Latin diets at:

www.e-guana.net/ organizations.php3?orgid=61&typeID= 193&action=printContentItem&itemID=1521

Asian People living in Japan, China, Taiwan, Korea, India, Vietnam, and other south Asian countries tend to eat a similar diet, one that researchers say is associated with lower rates of certain cancers, heart disease, and obesity. Here are the hallmarks of an Asian-style diet:

- Rice, rice products, noodles, breads, and grains (preferably whole) build the foundation of the diet.
- Large amounts of vegetables and fruits, legumes, nuts, and seeds are consumed. Protein in the diet comes from vegetable sources and legumes, such as soy and lentils.
- Moderate amounts of fish, shellfish, and low-fat dairy are eaten.

- People in these areas drink moderate amounts of alcohol.
- Minimal amounts of red meat, poultry, eggs, and sugar are consumed.

In the early 1990s, a study of more than 10,200 Chinese men and women, conducted by Cornell, Oxford, and the Chinese Academy of Preventative Medicine, showed that the rates of heart disease, breast cancer, osteoporosis, and obesity were much lower in rural China than in Western societies. The rural dwellers tended to eat the same diet their ancestors had eaten for thousands of years: one rich with plant-based foods, low in meats, and containing three times more fiber than the Western diet. When researchers looked at Chinese living in urban areas, however, the rates of heart disease, cancers, and other diseases increased, correlating with the increased consumption of a Western-type diet. Obesity rates were also much higher in urban areas. The study concluded that the gradual change from a plant-based rural diet to a Westernized meat-based diet had more impact on the development of disease than ethnic or genetic background.

GET PSYCHED

"The point is, we can really prevent disease. We can empower ourselves instead of relying so much on fate and physicians. I'm not saying that [my] recipes take the place of seeing a doctor. But diet is a predictor of health we can control."
—Nina Simonds, Asian cuisine expert, in Psychology Today's "Healing Foods," July/August 1999

People in Okinawa, Japan, have the longest life expectancy rates in the world: women in Okinawa have an average life expectancy of 86 and men 78. (In 2005, the Centers for Disease Control in Atlanta reported life expectancy rates of 80.1 years for U.S. women and 74.8 years for men, with an average of 77.6, a record.) The 25-year Okinawa Centenarian Study took a fascinating look at the role of diet and nutrition on longevity, obesity, and health. Researchers studied more than 600 people over the age of 100 living in Okinawa. They found that these centenarians followed a diet high in rice and grains, as well as vegetables, fruits, legumes, and particularly soy products. They consumed moderate amounts of alcohol and little red meat, but at least 3 servings of omega-3–rich fish, particularly salmon, tuna, and mackerel. They also participated in moderate amounts of exercise, kept up strong familial and friendship bonds, and were optimistic and easygoing. Researchers also noticed that younger Okinawans who'd adopted a more Western way of eating— increased levels of saturated fats—were experiencing higher rates of heart disease and cancer than their elders.

I'm hearing a lot of good things about soy. How can adding more of it to my diet improve my health?

"Soy protein, because it's plant-based, is low in cholesterol and low in satu- rated fats, unlike animal protein. Adding as little as one serving a day of soy can make a positive impact on your health. We've conducted several human trials that show adding soy to the diet significantly reduces total cholesterol. In one trial, there was a rise in HDL cholesterol–the good cholesterol–in women. And speaking of women, we did a six-month study with encouraging results that shows soy may protect against bone loss. However, we need to confirm that finding with studies lasting at least two years." *–John W. Erdman Jr., Ph.D., professor of nutrition, Department of Food Science and Human Nutrition, University of Illinois at Urbana-Champaign*

However, there are drawbacks to an Asian-style diet. For example, researchers note that segments of the population in Japan have a high rate of strokes, and they believe their higher consumption of sodium, along with a reduced consumption of fats and proteins, may be to blame. A diet high in sodium can lead to high blood pressure, a precursor to stroke, and the body needs fat and protein for healthy blood vessels. When blood vessels aren't healthy, there's more risk of stroke.

Following an Asian-style diet can be a good way to keep the pounds off while remaining healthy:

- Make whole-wheat pastas, brown rice, and whole grains the mainstay of your diet. Keep white rice and pasta to a minimum.
- Limit sodium intake. Ingredients such as soy and fish sauces are very high in sodium. At best, they'll make you retain water. At worst, a high-sodium diet puts you at risk for hypertension.
- Make high-fiber vegetables the focus of your meals rather than protein foods high in saturated fats.
- Substitute soy products for animal proteins.
- Limit the consumption of fried foods such as Chinese fried rice, Japanese tempuras, and Indian samosas.

Mediterranean We all know the French and Italians eat well. Studies show they, along with their other southern European neighbors, know how to stay healthy, too. Citizens of the countries in southern Europe, including Italy, Spain, Greece, Turkey, and southern France, tend to avoid the high coronary heart disease levels their northern neighbors suffer. They also tend to live longer, despite a relatively high-fat diet, in which fats make up 30 to 40 percent of their daily caloric intake.

The American Heart Association, which goes so far as to recommend a modified version of a Mediterranean diet, points out that there's no "one" Mediterranean diet. Many countries border the Mediterranean Sea, and all have individual histories, cultures, diets, and agricultural seasons. However, some commonalities exist in their diets:

- They're high in fruits, vegetables, breads and other cereals, potatoes, beans, nuts, and seeds.
- Olive oil provides an important source of monounsaturated fat, important for heart health.
- Dairy products, fish, and poultry are consumed in low to moderate amounts, while little red meat is consumed.
- Eggs are consumed zero to four times weekly.
- Wine is consumed in low to moderate amounts.

The first study touting the benefits of a Mediterranean-style diet was conducted in the 1950s by Ancel Keys, an epidemiologist who noticed that undernourished men in post-war Europe suffered less cardiovascular disease than their well-fed American counterparts. This observation led him to launch the Seven Countries Study in 1958. He and his team of researchers followed the diets, lifestyles, and heart health of more than 12,000 randomly selected men from the United States, Japan, Greece, Italy, the Netherlands, Finland, and the former Yugoslavia. Research eventually showed that heart disease was rare in men living in Mediterranean countries and Japan, where more heart-healthy unsaturated fats were consumed, versus the United States and Finland, where saturated fats played a greater role in the diet. Later in the study, Dr. Keys noted that lifestyle and physical activity were also factors contributing to coronary heart disease, but he contended that diet was the single most important factor in heart health. (It's interesting to note that Dr. Keys died in 2004, shortly before his 101st birthday.)

In another fascinating study conducted in the 1990s, doctors in Lyon, France, actually stopped a randomized, controlled trial testing the effectiveness of a Mediterranean diet on heart attack survivors. Halfway through the study, they noticed a 70 percent lower death rate within the experimental group—the men who were following a Mediterranean diet—and decided it would be unethical to allow the control group—men who were following a standard low-fat diet—to continue.

PsychSpeak

Metabolic syndrome is a group of metabolic risk factors that puts a person at risk for coronary heart disease, stroke, type 2 diabetes, and other health conditions. Risk factors include obesity, high triglyceride levels, low HDL cholesterol levels, and high blood pressure, among others. Many medical professionals question the syndrome as a distinct medical condition, however. More research is needed.

More recently, researchers in Italy conducted a randomized single-blind trial of a Mediterranean-type diet on 180 patients who had *metabolic syndrome* at a university hospital from 2001 to 2004. Ninety patients in the intervention group were instructed to follow the Mediterranean-style diet; the individuals received detailed instructions about what specific foods to eat. The 90 patients in the control group were instructed to follow a balanced diet consisting of 50 to 60 percent carbohydrates, 15 to 20 percent protein, and total fats of less than 30 percent.

After 2 years, patients who followed the Mediterranean diet had significant decreases in body weight, blood pressure, glucose levels, insulin, total cholesterol, and triglycerides, and a significant increase in levels of high-density lipoprotein (HDL) cholesterol, compared to the control group. Forty patients who followed the Mediterranean diet plan still showed features of metabolic syndrome, but 78 patients in the control group also had features. The overall prevalence of metabolic syndrome was reduced by approximately 50 percent in the intervention group. And here in the United States, another study conducted by Harvard Medical School and Brigham and Women's Hospital showed that adherence to a moderate-fat Mediterranean-style diet was easier for subjects than a low-fat diet, resulting in better weight-loss results.

With modifications, a Mediterranean-type diet can be used to lose weight:

- Consume less than 30 percent of your total calories from fat. Aim for 10 percent polyunsaturated fats, 15 percent monounsaturated fats, and as few saturated fats as possible.

- Add more poultry, fish, and game to your diet, and reduce your intake of red meat.

- Choose color. The hallmarks of Mediterranean cooking are the vibrant reds, deep yellows, and earthy greens of its vegetables, fruits, legumes, and grains. Limit consumption of foods that lack color, such as sugars, potatoes, pastas, rice, and bread. If you drink wine, pick red, which contains heart-healthy flavonoids, over white.

- Choose whole grains over processed. You can find many Mediterranean breads and pastas made of whole wheat, buckwheat, rye, and other nutritious grains.

What You Can Do

Lifestyle diets offer a lot of variety, as well as comfort, to some people who must lose weight. They offer a sense of familiarity. They support beliefs and world views. They usually don't focus solely on the goal of weight loss, but offer it as an additional benefit.

- ☐ Just as with adopting a regular weight-loss plan, losing weight takes commitment. Thoroughly investigate how your current eating plan has affected your weight, and decide what changes you can easily make. For example, if you're a vegetarian who eats a lot of cheese for protein, think of lower-calorie ways you can meet this need. Increase your consumption of beans and rice, for example. Add more calcium-fortified soy products, and consume more lower-fat cheeses.

☐ If you're thinking of making sweeping lifestyle changes— going macrobiotic as well as tackling an obesity problem— proceed carefully. Big lifestyle changes are hard enough to make without adding another layer of major change.

☐ As with restriction diets, pull the elements of what you need from a lifestyle diet. If you don't feel like giving up all meat but are fascinated with vegetarianism, try eating a few veg-only meals each week. Is macrobiotics appealing? Add sea vegetables and miso soups to your diet.

☐ Eat more foods from other cultures. Visit an ethnic market and look at the vegetables and grains. Talk to friends from those cultures about how they eat. Check out library books on Indian cooking or Asian cuisine.

☐ You don't have to give up foods such as cheese and wine, as the French have proved. What you need to watch is portion size. I talk about portioning later in the book, but for now, know that enjoying a glass of red wine in the evening or nibbling on a bit of Roquefort isn't what piles on the pounds—it's drinking the whole bottle and eating too much cheese along with bread and crackers.

Fad Diets

Their advertisements tempt us on late-night television. They tease us with their promises. This time you *will* lose the weight. You'll shed pounds easily. You won't even know you're dieting. You can eat as much as you want and still lose weight when you follow the plan. You study the before and after pictures of ordinary people, just like you, who've lost 20, 50, or more than 100 pounds on the diet, painlessly and easily. Or maybe the ads show you a celebrity who's struggled with her weight for years ... she's lost the weight by following this diet. Why not you?

After months or years of sacrifice, you feel yourself being swayed. As you reach for your credit card, you tell yourself, "Maybe there *is* a better and easier way of losing weight ..."

Americans spend nearly $33 billion each year on weight-loss products, including books, pills, and programs. Much of this money is spent on products that don't work. Nearly every dieter has tried some weight-loss fad—from chugging chalky-tasting shakes and eating grapefruit all day, to popping herbal supplements in hope that the fat will melt off overnight. A few pounds may come off with these eating schemes, but inevitably, when the diet ends, so does the weight loss. We learn nothing from the experience and return to our old eating habits, regaining the weight we lost—and then some.

The appeal of these diets is strong. Deep in our hearts we know losing weight isn't something that's going to happen overnight. But we keep holding out for a miracle because deprivation feels so bad and our need for immediate gratification is so deep. And people who develop weight-loss fads know this and craft their advertising messages accordingly.

"Most of the people I see who are battling their weight are dealing with a long-term problem," says Robert Kushner, M.D., medical director of the Wellness Institute of Northwestern Memorial Hospital in Chicago. "People approach their weight like it's an acute problem like a rash or sore thumb. At first it may improve with a fad diet, but obesity and overweight are long-term problems, so you need long-term solutions. You need to adopt something that fits, not only today, but two years from now."

Kushner's bottom line: "If you go on a diet avoiding foods or certain rules, it's a very low likelihood you'll be able to sustain long-term weight loss."

Determining Fact from Fad

Fad diet marketers do a terrific job convincing us they'll solve our weight-loss problems once and for all. They present compelling evidence their diets work, such as showing us dramatic before-and-after photos of successful dieters and citing some important-sounding studies that back up their claims. They can make their dietary theories sound perfectly scientific. "Fad diets are good at selling themselves," says Darwin Deen, M.D., professor of clinical family and social medicine at the Albert Einstein College of Medicine of Yeshiva University in Bronx, New York. "Dieters think they're getting something a good diet can't offer."

For example, in the 1980s, food combining was the rage, thanks to a popular diet book called *Fit for Life*. In it, authors Harvey and Marilyn Diamond claimed fruits should never be combined with proteins or starches because the body cannot digest different types of foods at once; the food ends up fermenting in the stomach and creating toxic wastes the body can't easily eliminate. This, they said, is the reason why people gain weight. This explanation sounded perfectly reasonable to a lot of dieters. And indeed, when they followed the *Fit for Life* diet, they ended up losing weight. It was convenient to give credit to food combining, but the real story is that they lost weight because the diet they ended up following was low in calories. There is no scientific evidence that food combining negatively or positively affects your digestion, nor is there evidence that improper food combining creates toxic-waste buildup in the body.

According to the Calorie Control Council, a nonprofit organization that represents manufacturers of low-calorie and low-fat foods, a fad diet ...

- Promises a quick fix or rapid weight loss.
- Singles out certain foods as being "bad" or "danger" foods.
- Recommends avoiding certain foods or combinations of foods.
- Draws simple conclusions from complex studies. Often bases conclusions on studies that have not been published in peer-reviewed, scientific journals.

> ## GET PSYCHED
>
> "Weight loss is a choice you have to make, and you have to keep making it over and over again. You don't have to be perfect at it, but you have to imperfect infrequently."
> —Darwin Deen, M.D., professor of clinical family and social medicine at the Albert Einstein College of Medicine

- Bases its theory on only one study.

- Recommends that certain products be bought to aid in weight loss.

- Makes recommendations to a broad base of people and does not recognize differences among those people.

- Goes against generally accepted medical advice from a variety of credible health professionals and organizations.

Be wary when you're faced with a weight-loss plan that sounds too good to be true. Like weight-loss diets in general, fad diets have high failure rates. But when you look at testimonials in ads for weight-loss shakes, for example, they'll include a disclaimer in small type that says, "Results not typical." This should give you some pause, especially if you're also hearing claims that the plan is easy to follow. If losing weight is so easy with these shakes, why aren't the results you're seeing typical?

Another tip-off to a possible rip-off is advertising that tells you to follow a sensible diet and exercise plan when you're using the product. If you follow a sensible diet and exercise plan, guess what? You're going to lose weight! You don't need to buy the product to achieve that end.

WEB TALK: Does a diet claim sound too good to be true? Check it out at the Quackwatch website at:
www.quackwatch.com

Many of these products and plans are very good at manipulating us into believing that "this time will be different." Part of our brain wants to believe we can lose weight without the hard work. Unfortunately, we usually end up disappointed and more frustrated with ourselves after we buy into the diet or product's claims. The cycle is insidious. The failure we experience on these supposedly "easy" plans becomes more psychological proof that we don't have what it takes to lose weight.

"Crash" Diets

"Lose 10 Pounds in Two Weeks!" the headline on a newsstand magazine screams. "The Amazing New Diet Your Doctor Won't Tell You About!" proclaims the cover of a diet book. "Turn your body into a fat-burning machine overnight with our weight-loss shakes!" the e-mail in your inbox promises. For many of us, these diet claims are irresistible. We end up starving ourselves for 2 weeks or gorging on grapefruit or parting with our hard-earned dollars for some chalky-textured "nutrition" shakes. And we do lose the weight. But then we kick ourselves, because when the diet ends, so does the weight loss—in fact, we're usually so hungry that we gain back all the weight we lost—plus some.

Crash diets have been around for years. Some of them, such as the infamous Cabbage Soup Diet, are still popular. All you do is eat cabbage soup for breakfast, lunch, and dinner, and voilà! Off comes the weight. Harvard-trained lawyer Susan Estrich even went so far as to recommend the Cabbage Soup Diet to jump-start her permanent weight-loss plan in her book, *Making the Case for Yourself: A Diet Book for Smart Women*.

Rapid-weight-loss diets tend to follow predictable patterns:

- They focus on a single food: cabbage soup; grapefruit; peanut butter; cider vinegar.
- They claim anyone can lose weight on the diet, no matter what their size, shape, sex, personality traits, or age.
- They promise fast results.
- They come with cute, catchy names such as "The Little Black Dress Diet" or "The Hollywood Diet."

And you know what? These crash diets *do* work. Almost anyone can lose weight and fit into a little black dress when all they eat for 2 weeks straight is cabbage soup.

Robert Kushner, M.D., medical director of the Wellness Institute at Northwestern Memorial Hospital in Chicago, points out that crash diets actually do have three benefits. The vast majority of these diets do result in weight loss. And as the weight comes off, the dieter may feel a sense of accomplishment. And finally, the experience shows the dieter he or she *can* lose weight, proving their body follows the laws of nature just like every other body.

It's not the crash diet's focus on a single food that causes weight loss. What causes the weight loss is a major reduction in daily caloric intake, usually to a number that's below the recommended daily intake for adults trying to lose weight. You can only eat so much cabbage soup in a day before it gives you uncomfortable intestinal gas. And let's face it, cabbage soup's not something you're going to sit down and pig out on. Grapefruit, on the other hand, possesses no mysterious fat-burning qualities, despite the hype. You could substitute other low-calorie fruits or

you're not alone

It started when I was 14 and I got dragged off to the doctor about my weight. He prescribed diet pills. Today, doctors do things a lot differently—they tell you how to eat healthily and urge you to exercise more. Back then, they gave you pills. I lost weight, but the pills made me sick. I had terrible headaches. I felt awful. And of course, the weight came back on when I stopped taking the pills.

Over the years I've gone on hundreds of diets. I must have joined Weight Watchers 50 times. I've done the Cabbage Soup Diet. I've done liquid diets, which made me feel like an alien from space. I've gone for psychiatry and hypnosis. I've even had acupuncture on my ears. Now I ask myself, "What was I thinking?"

veggies such as oranges, apples, or lettuce for the grapefruit and still lose the weight.

The problem with crash diets is that the 5-, 10-, or 20-pounds-at-best weight loss they create doesn't last. When you go on a crash diet, you tend to lose water weight. Dr. Kushner points out that crash diets are usually adhered to for days and weeks, not a lifetime. After the diet is discontinued and normal eating patterns resume, the weight returns.

Although Kushner doesn't endorse crash diets, he says there's very little danger following them, unless they're used excessively or the dieter has an underlying medical condition. Short-term complications might include bad breath, gas, headaches, constipation, lightheadedness, or fainting.

A steady diet of crash diets, however, is a different story. These diets are really all about severe calorie restriction, and we know how the human body responds to restriction (see Chapter 4). Because you're continually putting your body into feast-or-famine mode with these diets, you end up reinforcing that starvation-protection device evolution has created within your cells. That's why you tend to lose water weight on crash diets; when you're

I don't do the fad dieting anymore. Wisdom comes at middle age. My wakeup call was breast cancer. That, and I had my triglycerides checked—mine were in the very-high range. I decided weight loss wasn't the goal anymore—it was a healthier lifestyle.

I joined Weight Watchers again and took off 10 pounds. I never stop thinking I want to feel better, look better, and be healthier, because all those things equal losing weight. When I get discouraged, I remember the most important things in our lives don't come easily—why should losing weight be any different? Then I take another small step forward.

—*Donna, New York, New York*

taking in too few calories each day, your body defends against starvation. Water and protein are released from your body first, and fat is released only when absolutely necessary. Your metabolism slows, and it becomes more difficult to lose weight on your next diet because your body learns to use fewer calories to maintain your current weight.

Over-the-Counter Weight-Loss Supplements

It's tempting to believe a magic weight-loss pill will curb your appetite, speed up your metabolism, and burn fat while you sleep. Some of these over-the-counter (OTC) supplements do include ingredients that assist with those functions. But do they work long-term and are they safe? The answers to those questions aren't very heartening.

OTC weight-loss supplements are usually herb-based formulas, which are classed as "dietary supplements" by the Food and Drug Administration. Supplements don't fall under the same umbrella as, say, Meridia, a prescription weight-loss drug. Prescription drugs must be proven safe and effective for consumers before they can be legally dispensed. They are tested and retested until the FDA determines the drug is worthy of its approval.

This is not the case with dietary supplements. With these products, safety and effectiveness are determined by the manufacturer, not the FDA. Moreover, unlike drug manufacturers, supplement manufacturers are not required by law to report or forward to the government any complaints or claims they receive regarding illness or injury caused by their products. So when it comes to OTC weight-loss supplements, you're putting your faith—and possibly your health—in the manufacturer's hands.

WEB TALK: Find more up-to-date information about OTC weight-loss supplements at the NIH's Office of Dietary Supplements at:

➤ ods.od.nih.gov/

Because of an OTC weight-loss supplement called ephedra, the U.S. government is starting to come down a little harder on marketers who promise easy weight loss at the expense of health and well-being. Ephedra was one of the more well-known weight-loss supplements on the market a few years ago. The principle ingredient of ephedra is ephedrine, which when synthesized by the body performs much like a drug. Also known as ma huang or country mallow, ephedra was used by millions of dieters and athletes because it had an amphetaminelike effect on the nervous system—it speeds up metabolism. The herb was usually combined with caffeine, another nervous system stimulant. The combination effect was that it reduced appetite, allowing consumers to cut calories without feeling deprived. Dieters claimed the weight came off easier, and athletes believed it improved their sports performance.

Q&A

Can any herbal supplement on the market help me lose weight?

According to a November 2004 article in *American Family Physician*, the news on herbal remedies for weight loss looks discouraging. The three Harvard Medical School–based authors looked at the research on nearly 200 individual and combination formulations for weight loss, including the now-banned ephedra, as well as chromium, ginseng, guar gum, hydroxycitric acid, chitosan, and other products currently available to consumers. They concluded that the only product that showed a modest effect on weight loss was ephedra—and it's the one product that's illegal. The authors suggested family physicians discourage their patients from using any OTC weight-loss supplements because none met the criteria for recommended use.

But then the media started reporting ephedra's side effects. Some of them were minor: studies showed ephedra could cause heart palpitations, tremors, and insomnia. But other side effects were more frightening: strokes, heart attacks, and even death came to seemingly healthy consumers after they'd taken the supplement. Ephedra made headline news when it was linked to the death of Baltimore Oriole's pitcher Steve Bechler early in 2003.

Based on additional research and news reports about the supplement, in April 2004 the FDA made the sale of ephedra illegal in the United States, the first time it ever placed a market ban on an herbal supplement. The agency also promised it would keep a closer watch on other ingredients, such as bitter orange, aristolochic acid, and usnic acid, which are currently being used in OTC weight-loss formulations and are believed to be associated with liver and kidney problems.

Looking for a replacement for ephedra, weight-loss marketers figured out that bitter orange combined with caffeine provided a metabolic boost. The weight-loss from bitter orange isn't as dramatic as that from ephedra, and it's generally regarded as safe. Still, studies still need to be conducted on its long-term use for weight loss. In a 2004 review in *Experimental Biology and Medicine,* two Georgetown University researchers noted that Seville orange (*Citrus aurantium*) may have the potential to cause blood pressure and cardiovascular events because it contains synephrine, a bioactive substance that is structurally similar to epinephrine. The researchers also believe there's little evidence that bitter orange is really effective for weight loss. They noted there can be serious drug interactions and anyone who takes a regular medication should check with their doctor first before taking this supplement.

In November 2004, the Federal Trade Commission launched "Operation Big Fat Lie," a nationwide law-enforcement sweep designed to stop six companies from making false claims about their weight-loss products. Not only did the government agency file suit against the supplement marketers,

WEB TALK: Learn how to evaluate diet claims at:

www.ftc.gov/dietfit/

but they are also working with the media to help them reject unscrupulous advertising.

 The salesperson at a local supplement store told me their new proprietary weight-loss pills cause "thermogenesis." He guarantees I'll lose more weight faster and easier than before—and I can still eat my favorite foods. It sounds too good to be true.

It probably is. *FDA Consumer* says dieters should be very wary of any weight-loss supplement that …

- *Promises easy weight loss.* For most people, weight loss is only achieved through reducing calorie intake and increasing energy output.

- *Makes paranoid accusations.* Marketers will often claim the medical community puts down their products because the products threaten their standing. The FDA asks consumers to consider whether health professionals would really stand in the way of helping millions of patients.

- *Spouts meaningless medical jargon.* This impressive-sounding language often works as a smokescreen for lack of scientific proof.

If you have any questions at all about the effectiveness and safety of an OTC diet pill, check with your physician before you part with your cash.

(Courtesy of FDA Consumer, *November–December 1999)*

The government's stepped-up scrutiny of OTC supplement marketers is good news for consumers. But unless the laws change, marketers are still under no obligation to prove their weight-loss products are effective, never mind safe. The burden of proof falls on the government's shoulders to show these products are unsafe and ineffective. So you have to ask yourself: are you willing to put your health in the hands of someone who may only be thinking of his own bottom line?

Like crash dieting, herbal supplements are a short-term—and most likely, no-win—solution to a long-term weight-management issue.

you're not alone

I've always been aware of my weight. When I was a sophomore or junior in high school, I went to see my pediatrician about it. I lost about 15 pounds by dieting, but then I stopped and the weight came back on. That's when I turned to fast measures to take off the weight: I went to GNC and bought these pills. I took about 8 to 10 pills a day and wouldn't eat much, maybe a half an apple for lunch.

In college, I went on the *Fit for Life* plan. I had to buy these special bars and shakes; they were absolutely disgusting. I'd rather not eat than eat those bars. And there was one day where you could eat anything you wanted. That probably wasn't the best thing for my personality type.

After college I tried ephedra. The first time I took it, I took a stronger dose than I was supposed to. I remember I was at work and someone came up behind me and said my name. I jumped about 3 feet in the air because I was so wired. My heart was racing; I knew this wasn't good. So I tried Atkins. It was fun to have rules—you can eat this, but not that—but I was miserable on the diet. The turning point was when my boyfriend took me to an Italian restaurant and there was nothing on the menu I was "allowed" to eat.

My boyfriend and I quit smoking last year. It was an excuse for me to put on more weight. I'm an intelligent person—I knew it wasn't my knowledge of diet and exercise holding me back; it was me. I went to my M.D. and asked if she'd recommend a nutritionist and shrink. She sent me to Northwestern Memorial Hospital's Wellness Institute, where they have nutritionists, doctors, exercise specialists, and bariatric specialists on staff.

That's what it took for me. I learned that dieting is all about moderation. I've lost 25 pounds and kept it off. There aren't any "bad" foods. I was staying away from breads and sweets, but I've learned if I restrict something, I just want it more. My shrink instructed me to buy foods I didn't think I could have around, stuff like ice cream. She told me to eat one serving size every day— no more, no less, even if I didn't want it that day. It rewired me so those foods just aren't that special to me.

I can't believe it took me so long to figure all this out. My friends tell me I look great and that I seem different. People are faced with so many diets and so much food marketing, I wish they had more access to the how and why of losing weight like I did. I tell people to talk to their M.D.s ... they love it when patients are willing to talk to them about their weight. That's what they're there for. They can give you some options. —*Claire Z., 25, Chicago, Illinois*

Detox Diets and Fasting

Detox diets are built on the premise that weight gain and poor health are caused by excess toxins that build up in the human body. Followers of detox diets claim that poor dietary habits, improper food combining, and "bad foods" such as dairy and wheat clog up the body's digestive system. Some of these supposed toxins reside in our body for years, creating a habitat that makes it impossible for us to lose weight. The solution, thus, is to rid the body of these toxins through diet, herbal supplements, teas, or through more radical procedures such as colonic irrigation, where a tube is inserted into the rectum and the colon is washed out with water.

Detox diets have gained popularity in recent years. It's appealing for a lot of people to think that all they have to do is give the inside of their bodies a good spring cleaning and they'll lose weight. Or if they take the right herbal combinations and drink cleansing herbal teas, they'll force their liver and other organs to detoxify, thus making weight loss easier.

A variation on detox diets is fasting. Some fasting diets forbid food for a day or several days, but some allow juice. Other fasting diets allow water only. Advocates believe that fasting, like detox diets, will rid the body of toxins that prevent weight loss. They also claim fasting gives your digestive system a much-needed "rest." Some people who fast report feeling more in touch with their selves and their bodies.

But many others who've tried fasting feel nothing but a gnawing hunger. There's no medical evidence that fasting promotes weight loss better than a sensible diet combined with exercise. Generally, any weight lost on a fasting diet returns after the fast is over because fasting is basically a starvation diet. Fasting also deprives your body of essential nutrients your metabolism needs to perform effectively.

Robert Kushner, M.D., medical director of the Wellness Institute at Northwestern Memorial Hospital, dismisses weight-loss plans based on the detoxification concept. He admits the idea is appealing—that we can actually "clean out" years of accumulated gunk in our digestive systems—but he thinks the human body does a perfectly fine job with elimination. "When it comes to a detox diet," he says, "there are no positives. I can't think of any rationale to following a diet based on imagery or mysticism."

Like crash diets, you'll probably lose some weight on a detox diet or fast. The credit goes to a sharp reduction in caloric intake, however, not the magical combination of detoxifying herbs, juices, and foods, or the cleansing ability of a fast.

Strange-but-True Diets

Are you A, B, AB, or O? According to a diet book that came out recently, people should eat according to their blood types. Each type has "good" foods and "bad" foods that should be avoided. When you eat the right foods for your blood type, the book's author assures readers they'll lose weight.

Or dieters can look to the stars to figure out what they should be eating to stay healthy and lose weight. The astrological sign diet will tell you not only what you should eat, but how your sun sign copes with weight loss. If you're a Scorpio, rejoice! Rapid weight loss is easier for you than any other sign. If you're a Libra, bad luck—the stars say you have a slow metabolism and put weight on easily.

And I've already mentioned food combining, a diet popular in the 1980s. This eating plan comes with a long list of rules: don't eat proteins with starches, consume fruit on an empty stomach, etc. Weight loss occurs only when certain foods are eaten at the right time of day and in the proper combinations.

The problems with diets like these are many. First, there's no scientific evidence that eating according to blood type, astrological signs, or food combinations promotes weight loss. Second, although you may lose weight on these plans, it's not because your blood type has been accommodated, your dietary stars were in alignment, or your apple was consumed on an empty stomach. You lose weight on fad diets like these because they tend to be low in calories. Rather than focus on sound nutritional principles, however, they rely on scientifically unsound food rules that take no consideration of your personality, motivations, or preferences.

Bottom line, according to Kushner: "I can't think of any logical way how these diets will lead to any good."

Celebrity-Endorsed Diets

Remember when Oprah Winfrey dropped 70 pounds in 1988? According to an article in *Time* magazine, when Oprah gave credit to Optifast on her television show, the diet company was bombarded with 200,000 telephone calls from viewers hours after her show aired. Five years later, Oprah introduced her fans to her personal chef, Rosie Daley, who was credited with helping the star keep her weight down. Daley ended up writing a diet-friendly cookbook, *In the Kitchen with Rosie: Oprah's Favorite Recipes,* which went on to sell more than 6 million copies in hardcover.

Americans are star-struck when it comes to dieting. And it's no wonder. We love peeking into the lives of the rich and famous. Popular television shows such as *Newlyweds: Nick and Jessica* and *The Osbournes* deliver these stars into our living rooms. We snap up magazines such as *People, US Weekly, Star,* and *National Enquirer* to learn how Jennifer Aniston slims down (the Zone) and J-Lo keeps her booty up. With a twist of schadenfreude, we devour stories about stars who struggle with their weight. By the same token, we believe if we follow another celebrity's diet plan, we can earn a measure of what she has: a slim body, good looks, and glamour.

Weight Watchers hired Sarah Ferguson, the Duchess of York, to act as its spokesperson. Jenny Craig has Kirstie Alley as its spokesperson. Some celebrities have actually turned into diet book authors, taking the cult of celebrity to a new level. Suzanne Somers, the former *Three's Company* television star, has penned several diet books and actually has a diet named after her: Somersizing. Marilu Henner, another popular television actress, wrote a diet book called *Total Health Makeover*, which urged readers to forego all sugar and dairy products. Tough-talking television host Dr. Phil admonished the overweight to "get real" in his diet book and even markets nutritional supplements, shakes, and nutrition bars to go along with his plan. More recently, model Carol Alt has jumped on the celebrity diet bandwagon with her book, *Eating in the Raw,* which touts the benefits of a raw food diet.

Celebrities add a sense of legitimacy to a diet, according to Robert Kushner, M.D. They become diet authorities by virtue of their celebrity. We'll overlook the fact that they don't have expertise in nutrition because we admire their fame, their figures, their looks. Or as in Dr. Phil's case, we accord them admiration for their charisma, power, and a reputation for telling it like it is. It's human nature to want these same qualities in ourselves, so we're willing to fork over our money to experience them.

When you're tempted to follow the diet your favorite star swears by or you're considering an eating plan touted by one of these celebrity-turned-diet-counselors, keep several things in mind:

No matter how closely you follow the diet, you're never going to look like the celebrity who's endorsing it. Looking good is a full-time job for a lot of these people—what you're seeing in books and magazines is not only the results of the diet, but also the team results of makeup artists, hairdressers, stylists, trainers, lighting specialists, and even touch-up artists.

Celebrity does not equal knowledge. They may know how to act, model, or build a multimillion-dollar television enterprise, but that doesn't give them the edge on nutrition.

Be skeptical about what you read. Many magazines will print "celebrity diet issues" that claim insider knowledge about how stars keep in shape. These "scoops" can come from anywhere— from a publicist wishing to keep a client's book in the news to a Hollywood fitness trainer eager for PR.

You have to choose a diet plan that makes sense for *you*. Good for your favorite star if she can stay healthy by eating a macrobiotic diet, doing yoga 2 hours a day, and working out with a trainer. But this is probably not a diet and exercise plan you'll be able to stick to, never mind afford. Better to look for diet solutions you can apply to your life today.

This isn't to say every celebrity who writes a diet book is out to take advantage of their fame. A good example is Sarah Ferguson, the Duchess of York, who continues to work with Weight Watchers and has even written a few books under the Weight Watchers brand. Ferguson was ridiculed in the British press during her marriage to Prince Andrew for her fluctuating weight. Upon their divorce, Ferguson finally gave up the yo-yo dieting and learned to manage her weight through Weight Watchers, one of the more sensible diet plans out there. Yes, she gets paid by the organization, but on the other hand, she's walked the walk. Anyone who's struggled with their weight or been compared to a prettier, more fit relative can identify with her. On top of this, she has an organization backing her that is respected by many diet experts and medical professionals for its weight-loss successes.

> ## GET PSYCHED
>
> "The [Duchess of York] is a role model. She creates inspiration for people because she is so candid, so interesting, so willing to talk openly about weight, that it makes it OK for others to do the same."
> —Linda Webb Carilli, R.D., Weight Watchers spokesperson, quoted in Psychology Today, January/February, 2002

What You Can Do

Take heart. Although there may be no easy or fast way for you to lose weight, there's no fast or easy way for anyone else to, either. Weight loss is hard work for everyone, whether they're young, old, rich, poor, unknown, or famous. But remember—weight loss isn't all about hardship and deprivation. You'll find plenty of rewards on your weight-loss journey if you remain focused on making incremental changes rather than get-fixed-quick solutions.

❑ Remember, if it sounds too good to be true, it usually is. Remain skeptical of any diet or product that makes weight loss sound effortless and easy.

☐ Thoroughly research any weight-loss technique, system, supplement, or diet you consider. What do medical experts say about it? Are there any safety concerns?

☐ If you decide to take an OTC weight-loss supplement, check with your doctor first, especially if you have other health conditions besides overweight or obesity.

☐ Report any adverse effects of supplements, teas, or other weight-loss products to your doctor. Ask your doctor to report the incident to the FDA's Med Watch hotline at 1-800-FDA-1088 (1-800-332-1088). You may also report the incident yourself at www.fda.gov/medwatch/report/consumer/consumer.htm.

☐ Consider taking dietary and weight-loss advice only from trained health-care professionals who know you personally, so you can be sure you're getting the best advice tailored to your needs.

☐ Remember that anyone who spends his or her life in the limelight also spends a lot of time working on looking good. There's nothing wrong with this, except it can be hard to hold yourself to the same standard. Take what you can use from these role models, and don't agonize over what you can't.

Clinically Supervised Weight Loss

For many Americans, there comes a day when losing weight stops being an option and turns into a grave necessity. Weight loss is no longer about fitting into a size 12. Exercise stops being something you'll do someday when you find the time.

The turning point can be dramatic. It's a 60-year-old man looking forward to retirement learning from his doctor he's diabetic. It's a severely obese 35-year-old mother of three young children being told she exhibits four symptoms of metabolic syndrome. It's a 45-year-old businessman who's suffered a major heart attack, really listening to his doctor for the first time. They are all hearing, "You're one of the lucky ones. You can still make changes. But you've got to make them soon or else ...."

You may have heard them yourself. They're scary words to hear, and you might be feeling unlucky. You can't put off weight loss anymore. Years of overweight have caught up to you, and it's time to pay the piper. You have a lot of questions. Do you have to radically change your lifestyle? Will you ever be able to eat like a normal person? If you haven't been able to lose weight before, how can you possibly lose it now? And how can you manage weight loss when you may have a serious health concern besides overweight and obesity to consider? Can your health get any worse?

Millions of Americans every year turn poor health around through a sound weight-loss plan and moderate exercise—and you can, too. You have an opportunity to make changes.

Why You May Need More Diet Supervision

If you have a significant amount of weight to lose or you have other medical problems compounding your overweight and obesity, it's important to work with a medical professional. They're going to know your individual health history, what your risks are, and what type of program will work best for you.

A medically supervised weight-loss plan is recommended for a young child or adolescent—or someone who's at the other end of the age spectrum. A diet can put a lot of physiological stress on the body. The body of a relatively healthy, yet overweight

you're not alone

It was the summer after my college graduation. I wasn't feeling very well, so I went to see my primary care doctor. He checked me over and said, "Well, it's no wonder—you weigh 239 pounds and your blood pressure is 150/90." He put me on anti-hypertensive medications, basically diuretics. He told me to come back and see him every month to weigh in, and he'd write down my weight in my file. Let's just say that the power of the white lab coat definitely made an impact.

I was starting a job in Washington and commuting from Baltimore every day. I was working like a farmer, up at the crack of dawn and getting home after the sun had set. I only had about 2 hours of free time every day. You can only eat so much in just 2 hours. Between the looming authority figure of my doctor and the travails

adult can handle this stress, but in someone young or old, a diet should be monitored.

When you're carrying around excess weight, you're also prone to developing conditions such as high blood pressure (hypertension), high cholesterol levels, heart disease, type 2 diabetes, breathing problems, sleep apnea, arthritis, and some forms of cancer. The research on the link between obesity and these serious conditions is sobering; some 70 percent of people who become severely overweight also develop at least one of these *comorbidities*. If you are dealing with excess weight, as well as a condition such as heart disease, simply following the latest diet trend may have serious consequences for your health. A weight-loss plan that includes medical supervision is the best course of action for you.

PsychSpeak

A **comorbidity** is a co-existing or additional condition or disease that affects another condition or disease, in this case, obesity. Comorbidities can cause additional challenges or health problems for obese patients to overcome.

and nervous tension of working in D.C., I dropped over 40 pounds in a few months. Because I needed to get my blood pressure down, I cut back on salt by doing away with the salt shaker. I simply used salt substitute and Mrs. Dash spices on food. And I started eating less food, took walks in the morning, and rode my stationary bike. It was the last 20 pounds that were the toughest to come off, but I kept at it.

Today, I feel I am much more the person I was meant to be. I'm more confident, outgoing, and I take pride in myself. Family and friends used to say that I would be a handsome guy if I just did something about the weight. And now, well, I'm told that I am and I feel that I am, both inside and out. –*Dan Collins, 42, Baltimore, Maryland*

Q&A

What is waist-to-hip ratio, and why should I be concerned about it?

Waist-to-hip ratio is a measurement of body shape that reveals whether you're at risk for some serious conditions. It is calculated by dividing the waist measurement by the hip measurement. Research shows that people who put on fat in their midsections versus their hips and thighs are more likely to develop heart disease and diabetes. These people tend to have deposits of fat, called visceral or intra-abdominal fat, around vital organs. Researchers aren't quite sure why this kind of fat is so bad for one's health; one theory is that visceral fat secretes fatty acids near the liver which causes disease.

To figure out waist-to-hip ratio: a female with a 42-inch waist measurement divided by a 45-inch hip measurement has a waist-to-hip ratio of .93. A male with a 50-inch waist and a 42-inch hip measurement has a waist-to-hip ratio of 1.19.

For men, a ratio of .90 or less is considered safe. For women, a ratio of .80 or less is considered safe. For both men and women, a ratio of 1.0 or higher is considered "at risk" or in the danger zone. Osama Hamdy, M.D., Ph.D., director of the Obesity Clinic at Harvard's Joslin Diabetes Center and an instructor at Harvard Medical School, points out that someone who is slim but carries excess weight in the belly area may also be at risk for developing chronic health conditions.

The great news is that there's strong evidence that weight loss, exercise, and lifestyle modification can make a positive impact on many, if not all, of these health conditions. When one problem is solved (the weight loss), the other problems (the high blood pressure, the breathing problems) may resolve themselves, too, or the weight loss might at least help these other problems. Sometimes all you need is a caring health professional who can guide you toward the right changes in your life. For other people, a more aggressive action plan for weight loss is necessary.

Q & A

What is metabolic syndrome?

Metabolic syndrome (also called syndrome x) is a group of metabolic risk factors that put a patient at risk for developing coronary heart disease, other diseases related to plaque buildup in artery walls, and type 2 diabetes. It is closely linked to insulin resistance, which is why it is often called the insulin resistance syndrome. The American Heart Association estimates that 47 million adults in the United States have metabolic syndrome.

According to the Third Report of the National Cholesterol Education Program (NCEP) Expert Panel on Detection, Evaluation, and Treatment of High Blood Cholesterol in Adults (Adult Treatment Panel III), metabolic syndrome is identified by the presence of three or more of these components:

- Central obesity as measured by waist circumference; for men, 40 inches or more; for women, 35 inches or more

- Fasting blood triglycerides greater than or equal to 150 mg/dL

- Blood HDL cholesterol for men of 40 mg/dL or less and women of 50 mg/dL or less.

- Blood pressure greater than or equal to 130/85 mmHg

- Fasting glucose greater than or equal to 110 mg/dL

Medical professionals agree the safest and most effective way to reduce characteristics of metabolic syndrome in overweight and obese people is by losing weight and increasing physical activity.

Clinical Weight-Loss Options

The big difference between a clinical weight-loss program and your local commercial weight-loss center is that the clinical program is staffed by trained health-care and/or mental health professionals. A commercial weight-loss center may have doctors, nutritionists, researchers, and psychologists working for it, but they're usually not working on the front lines with dieters. When you're in a clinical program, you have some, if not exclusive, direct contact with physicians, psychiatrists, psychologists, registered dieticians, exercise physiologists, and nursing staff. This isn't to say a commercial weight-loss program is inferior to a clinical program. But for someone who needs more medical supervision because of their health history or who has psychological issues that run a little deep, a clinical program may be a good option.

Clinical weight-loss programs can be just like commercial weight-loss programs in that they are often run as a business. It can be a physician-run clinic that administers commercial liquid diets or a bariatric surgery practice. Other programs are affiliated with colleges, universities, and hospitals where profit takes a backseat to research gathering.

Moreover, there is no one type of clinical weight-loss program. It can be tailored to the slightly overweight or open only to the severely obese (BMI higher than 40). It can be a 12-week free program at your local hospital, open to anyone who is overweight.

PsychSpeak

Behavior modification is a technique for promoting the frequency of desirable behaviors and decreasing the incidence of unwanted ones.

Or it can be a pricey 3-month stay at one of the top hospitals in the United States. It may be supervised by an M.D. who prescribes very-low-calorie diets (VLCDs) or a psychologist who specializes in *behavior modification*. Or it can be run as a wellness center, where all aspects of weight loss— diet, exercise, nutrition, behavior, and lifestyle changes—are encouraged.

Clinical weight-loss programs tend to fall in one of four categories. Programs affiliated with universities and hospitals fall into the first category. These programs work with overweight and/or obese patients to help them acquire healthy eating habits and behavioral changes without prescribing a diet or surgery. Clinicians work with a person to make changes based on his or her specific needs, and the program development is based on proven research.

The second type of clinical program specializes in very low-calorie diets (VLCDs). These programs are supervised by medical professionals. VLCDs are commercially prepared liquid diets that usually consist of no more than 800 calories per day. The dieter eats no food on this diet and thus must be monitored in a clinical situation. A VLCD is recommended only for someone who is obese, not merely overweight.

The third type of clinical program prescribes weight-loss drugs to its patients. Like VLCD programs, prescription drugs are only appropriate for patients with significant amounts of weight to lose.

The fourth type of clinical program is *bariatric* or gastric surgery. Gastric surgery is usually the last resort for someone who is severely obese. This is a course of action for someone who has tried everything else and simply cannot lose weight. Although surgery is a drastic measure, patients tend to lose weight quickly and improve their health greatly.

PsychSpeak

Bariatrics is a branch of medicine that deals with the cause, prevention, and treatment of obesity.

There can be crossover among the four types of programs. You may find a university-based weight-loss program that also offers bariatric surgery for the severely obese. Some programs are run by psychologists and registered dieticians who are not affiliated with a university or hospital. Whatever clinical program you join, it should teach you the eating and exercise changes you'll need to adopt for the rest of your life. No matter if you take diet drugs, lose weight on a medically supervised liquid diet, or get gastric surgery, you'll need to make behavioral changes to help you keep the weight off forever.

University and Hospital Weight-Loss Programs

Many top hospitals and universities across the United States sponsor weight-loss and obesity programs. If you're lucky enough to live near one, a program such as this can be highly effective in helping you lose weight, changing your eating behaviors, and working with you to maintain weight loss. And if you don't live nearby, a few programs actually offer accommodations for a long-term stay.

Elena M. Ramirez, Ph.D., a licensed psychologist-doctorate, is director of the University of Vermont's Weight Control Program, an 18-week program for people who have a substantial amount of weight to lose. Ramirez identifies two types of weight-control programs, both research-based. One is a weight-control program that has been shown to work. The other conducts research to show that a weight-control program works. These programs collect data from participants for the purpose of strengthening weight-control treatments in the future. Programs designed to gather research usually have specific criteria for people joining the program. Sometimes researchers only want participants of a certain age or sex; other times participants who have certain psychological or health history backgrounds may be ruled out.

WEB TALK: If you're interested in participating in a research weight-loss program, check out what's available at:

▲ www.clinicaltrials.gov

Sometimes the research-based programs, such as Ramirez's, may collect data on participants or run studies, so there can be crossover between these two types of programs.

These weight-loss programs often put the word out to near-by doctors and hospitals that they're looking for participants. A common denominator among the people who join is that they've tried a lot of different diet programs in the past with disappointing results. One of the reasons why a research-based program is attractive is because it usually offers more personal support than a commercial plan. For example, Ramirez thinks Weight Watchers is an effective program for many dieters, but some people need more accountability. "At Weight Watchers, for example, you can be more anonymous," she says. "You can avoid the scale. You can decide not to show up for a meeting. But a program like ours is a little more personal. If they stop showing up, we start asking why and work with them to overcome any psychological obstacles they're having. We can work on some behavioral changes."

Ramirez advises prospective participants to look for the following when selecting a university-based weight-control program:

- Understand what kind of program you're getting into. There's a difference between a hospital or university program that uses research to help participants lose weight and a program that uses participants to gather research.

- Check out who's in charge. Some programs have students who work on the program, and that's fine. But Ramirez says at a minimum, a registered dietician and a psychologist should head the program. An exercise physiologist is also an important asset to a program.

- If you're joining a research-based program, look at the research attached to it. The program's philosophy should derive from empirical research and have outcome data that shows results.

Fees for programs such as these range from no cost to participants to a significant expense, especially if you're attending a long-term in-patient program. Sometimes health insurance picks up part of the cost; most of the time, however, the expense is all yours. Check with your doctor or call a local hospital or a university's community relations department to find programs near you. A number of hospital and university-based weight-loss programs are listed in Appendix C at the back of this book.

Very Low-Calorie Diets (VLCD)

Oprah Winfrey put liquid diets back on the map when she lost 80 pounds on the Optifast diet in the late 1980s. Optifast, as well as other liquid diets, is considered a very-low-calorie diet (VLCD), which is a commercially prepared formula of about 800 calories that replaces all foods for weeks or possibly months. VLCDs are designed to promote rapid weight loss for patients who are moderately to severely obese—usually someone with a BMI higher than 30—and, thus, are only to be used under medical supervision. Sometimes they're prescribed for patients with lower BMIs, but only if they have significant comorbidities that accompany overweight. VLCDs are not recommended for use by pregnant or breast-feeding women, young children, or adolescents. To reach maximum effectiveness, VLCDs should be part of a treatment that might include nutritional and exercise counseling, behavior modification, and/or prescription drug therapy.

When you're on a VLCD, you can expect to lose 3 to 5 pounds per week, or 44 pounds over 16 weeks. This kind of weight loss can improve conditions such as type 2 diabetes, high blood pressure, and high cholesterol levels, which makes the diet attractive for people who need to do something fast to change their health.

The bad news: weight gain is common after a VLCD. The National Institute of Diabetes and Digestive and Kidney Diseases says these diets may be no more effective than a diet based on dietary restriction. In a study published in the *Journal of the American Dietetic Association* in 2002, researchers wanted to determine what lifestyle, diet, and exercise factors prevented long-term weight regain after completion of a VLCD. Twenty-seven women who completed a VLCD program were studied 3 years later. Looking at food and exercise records as well as lifestyle questionnaires, researchers analyzed what led to weight-loss maintenance. They concluded that the women who limited intake of dietary fat and performed physical activity kept off the most weight.

Still, while weight loss on a VLCD can be dramatic, the diet itself is far less costly or physically altering than bariatric surgery. Anyone who goes on this diet will need to commit to dietary and exercise changes to maintain permanent weight loss.

Prescription Weight-Loss Medications

Another option for patients who must lose weight and lose it fast is to take prescription weight-loss medications. These drugs are recommended only for patients who are at risk for serious medical conditions because of their weight. They're approved for patients with BMIs higher than 30, or BMIs of 27 or above if they have comorbidities with their overweight, including high blood pressure or type 2 diabetes.

Weight-loss medications lead to an average weight loss of 5 to 22 pounds more than a dieter may lose with a nonsupervised diet. Maximum weight loss usually occurs within 6 months of beginning treatment and tends to stall or decrease during the remainder of the treatment. One of the reasons why prescription therapy is recommended for some patients is that short-term health gains can be good. Studies show that some patients who lose weight have improved blood pressure, blood cholesterol and triglyceride levels, and insulin resistance.

The biggest drawback with prescription weight-loss medications is that few studies have been conducted on their safety or effectiveness. When the drugs are taken short-term, the weight seems to come back after treatment is stopped, but new research suggests when the drugs are taken over the long term, weight loss may be maintained. The problem is that the drugs haven't been approved for long-term use, so more studies are needed to determine the drugs' effects. Moreover, all prescription weight-loss medications currently on the market are classified as controlled substances, except orlistat. If you have a history of alcohol or drug abuse, you should use caution in taking these drugs, although abuse and dependence with nonamphetamine appetite-suppressant drugs are not common.

According to a 2004 report released by the Health and Human Service's Agency for Healthcare Research and Quality, some prescription weight-loss medicines—specifically orlistat and sibutramine—are known to promote moderate weight loss when taken along with a sensible diet. The amount of weight lost directly attributable to the drugs averages less than 11 pounds, but even such a modest loss in weight may decrease the chance of developing type 2 diabetes. The review further showed that no weight-loss drug was superior to another, and, like all medications, each drug has side effects.

Prescription weight-loss drugs are most effective when they're combined with a healthful eating and exercise plan. Many insurance plans don't cover the cost of prescription diet drugs; they can be quite expensive if you're paying for them out of your own pocket.

Sibutramine *Brand name:* Meridia

Sibutramine is one of the more commonly prescribed appetite suppressants in the United States, along with phentermine. An appetite suppressant works by stimulating the appetite control center in the brain and affecting levels of neurotransmitters that make the patient feel less hungry and/or more full.

Sibutramine is approved by the FDA for 1 year of use. It's not a long-term solution to permanent weight loss. It is usually prescribed to patients who have a BMI higher than 30, or those with a BMI higher than 27 who have comorbidities with their overweight.

Side effects of sibutramine include increases in blood pressure and heart rate. People with blood pressure problems, heart disease, an irregular heartbeat, or a history of stroke should avoid sibutramine. Your doctor should also monitor your blood pressure regularly.

Orlistat *Brand name:* Xenical

Orlistat is known as a lipase inhibitor, which reduces the body's ability to absorb dietary fat. It blocks an enzyme called lipase, which is responsible for breaking down fats. When fats cannot be broken down, the body can't absorb them, so they pass through the body and are eliminated through bowel movements.

Again, people who take this drug must follow a low-calorie diet and perform regular exercise. It's safe to use for up to 2 years, but when the drug is discontinued, patients need to follow a diet and exercise plan that maintains the weight they've lost.

The side effects of a lipase inhibitor such as orlistat can be distasteful, especially if the patient insists on eating a diet high in fats. They may be plagued with gas that includes oily discharge, as well as an increased number of bowel movements, an urgent need to have them, and an inability to control them, particularly after high-fat meals are consumed. Not only does the drug block dietary fat from being absorbed, but it may also block the absorption of some vitamins, which is why a daily multivitamin is recommended to patients.

Phentermine *Brand name:* Adipex-P, Anoxine-AM, Fastin, Ionamin, Obephen, Obermine, Obestin-30, Phentrol

Phentermine is the other half of the fen-phen weight-loss pill, which the FDA pulled off the market in 1997 because of its link to cardiac valve disease. Phentermine, an appetite suppressant like sibutramine, is still approved for use in weight loss. Most patients take the drug for 4 to 6 weeks—it is a drug that should only be taken for short-term use. Side effects are rare but include dry mouth, unpleasant taste, diarrhea, constipation, and vomiting. It is not recommended for patients who have high blood pressure, heart disease, overactive thyroid, or glaucoma.

Other Prescription Weight-Loss Medications Physicians often prescribe to their patients other drugs not specifically developed for weight loss. This is called *off-label use*. Some such drugs include the following:

PsychSpeak

Off-label use is the practice of prescribing medication for periods of time or medical conditions not approved by the FDA. The FDA only regulates how a medication can be advertised or promoted by a manufacturer; it does not place any restrictions on a physician prescribing it.

- Antidepressants. Bupropion (Wellbutrin), which is FDA-approved for depression and smoking cessation, has been shown to help patients lose weight and maintain weight loss for up to 1 year.

- Seizure medications. Topiramate and zonisamide, which are used to treat seizures in epileptics, have been shown to help with weight loss.

- Diabetic medications. Metformin may help obese patients with type 2 diabetes lose small amounts of weight. It isn't clear how the drug works, but it does seem to reduce hunger and food intake in patients.

- Drug combinations. Researchers are also looking at drug combinations such as fluoxetine (brand name Prozac, an anti-depressant) with phentermine, and orlistat with sibutramine. But much research still needs to be done on the effectiveness and side effects of combining drugs.

- Drugs in development. Some of the more-promising drugs include rimonabant, which affects brain chemicals, and ciliary neurotrophic factor (CNTF), which is found in certain brain cells and affects appetite control hormones. These medications are currently only available in clinical trials.

Bariatric Surgery

When someone who is struggling with obesity has tried everything to lose weight—diets, commercial weight-loss programs, medically supervised diets—and can't lose the weight, bariatric surgery can be their lifesaver. Bariatric surgery has become more mainstream since celebrities such as Al Roker and Carnie Wilson underwent surgeries and went public with their stories. It is estimated that from 1993 to 2003, the number of gastric bypass surgeries rose more than 500 percent. In 2003, 103,200 Americans underwent bariatric surgery procedures, and in 2004, the American Society for Bariatric Surgery (ASBS) estimated the number increased to 140,000 Americans.

The decision to pursue bariatric surgery isn't one that can be taken lightly. In fact, when you visit a bariatric surgeon or specialist to discuss the procedure, you will be thoroughly tested. You'll have to exhibit certain physical requirements for initial consideration. After that, you'll be asked to meet with a psychologist for a mental health examination. Only when your doctor deems you mentally ready and physically capable of handling the operation will you be approved for surgery.

The National Institutes of Health says you may be a candidate for surgery if you have a body mass index (BMI) of 40 or more and are about 100 pounds overweight for men and 80 pounds for women.

GET PSYCHED

"All my life I dreamed of living a normal life. I get to now. It's no longer a dream." —Kirk T., Ohio, who lost 450 pounds through bariatric surgery

You might also be a candidate if you have a BMI between 35 and 39.9 and have a serious obesity-related health problem such as type 2 diabetes, heart disease, or severe sleep apnea. It's important that you also have an understanding of the operation and the lifestyle changes you will need to make.

Russell LaForte, M.D., director of the Center for Weight Management at the University of Texas at Galveston Medical Branch, says surgeons may have requirements the patient needs to meet beyond these basic requirements. Some doctors insist patients pass a psychological evaluation with a psychologist or psychiatrist before being approved for surgery. LaForte wants to see a patient who has exhausted all other routes to weight loss. "We get people who come into our practice and say, 'My neighbor Jane got the surgery and she looks great, so I want it, too.' It can't be entered into in a flippant manner."

Gastric surgery creates weight loss through food restriction and/or malabsorption. Restriction delays the amount of food that can be consumed, thus slowing the digestive process. Food cannot move quickly from the stomach into the small intestine. This creates a quick, long-lasting feeling of fullness in the patient; the patient simply can't eat any more until the stomach is emptied. Malabsorption happens when sections of the small intestine are bypassed by surgery. Only small amounts of nutrients get absorbed by the body; the rest of the undigested food matter passes into the large intestine and is moved out of the body. Some gastric surgery procedures use both of these methods to produce weight loss.

As with any surgery, gastric bypass procedures do have risks. Approximately 10 to 20 percent of surgery patients require follow-up surgeries to correct complications. Abdominal hernias are the most common complications; less common are breakdowns in the staple lines and stretched stomach outlets (stomas). More than one third of surgery patients develop gallstones because during rapid weight loss, the bile in the liver thickens, creating suscepti-bility to stones. To avoid this complication, many surgeons opt to remove the gallbladder during surgery as well. Nearly 30 per-cent of surgery patients develop nutritional deficiencies, such as anemia, osteoporosis, and metabolic bone disease. Women should avoid pregnancy until their weight becomes stable because nutri-tional deficiencies can hurt the fetus. The federal government reports that less than 1 percent of bariatric surgery patients die as a result of the surgery or from complications when they're per-formed by experienced surgeons.

The people who undergo bariatric surgery often have no other options. A report issued in 2004 by the Agency for Healthcare Research and Quality concluded that weight-loss surgery for ex-tremely obese patients who've tried everything else to lose weight may be more effective than drugs for people with BMIs of 35 to 40. Doctors say surgery is successful when 50 percent of the extra weight is lost and kept off for at least 5 years.

Bariatric surgery isn't cheap. The average procedure runs any-where from $20,000 to $35,000. In 2004, Medicare removed language from its Medicare Coverage Issues Manual that said obe-sity was not a disease, which opens the door for coverage of sur-gery. Some insurance companies pay for the procedure if a doctor deems the surgery medically necessary. But in 2005, more insurance companies around the country are declining to offer coverage because they believe they are seeing more unnecessary and unsafe surgeries. As a result, lawmakers in many states are trying to decide whether to pass legislation to make insurance companies pay for these procedures.

The Sapala-Wood Micropouch With the Sapala-Wood Micropouch procedure, the top of the stomach is completely divided. The division creates a small "micropouch," separate from the lower part of the stomach. The pouch ends up being the size of a grape, holding only 1 to 2 ccs of food.

Then the small intestine is divided into two pieces. One piece is connected with the pouch, and the other piece is connected to the distal small intestine to complete the circuit. When food is ingested, it passes through the esophagus, the pouch, and then to the intestine, bypassing the lower part of the stomach. This part of the stomach no longer receives any food or liquids, but it's still functional because the nerves and blood supply are left intact.

The Sapala-Wood Micropouch surgery greatly controls food intake because the pouch only holds 1 to 2 ccs of food. The anatomy becomes less susceptible to ulcers, and the procedure also limits the number of calories that can be absorbed by the GI tract. However, the surgery narrows or blocks the stomach, and vomiting can occur when food isn't properly chewed or is eaten too quickly.

Adjustable Gastric Banding With an adjustable gastric banding (AGB) procedure, a silicone elastomer band is placed around the upper end of the stomach to create a pouch that can only hold a small amount of food. The band creates a small opening where food can pass into the lower part of the stomach. It's unlike the Sapala-Wood Micropouch in that the lower part of the stomach still digests food. With this procedure, food moves into the lower stomach slowly, thus creating a feeling of fullness in the patient.

A small, hollow tube encircles the inside of the silicone elastomer band; the other end of the tube runs to a self-sealing access port just below the skin beneath the rib cage. This allows the band's circumference to be adjusted after surgery. A physician can inflate or deflate the tube with saline solution to adjust the stoma diameter in an outpatient setting.

This laparoscopic surgery is considered simple and relatively safe. Because laparoscopic surgery is minimally invasive, there's a short recovery period and complications are rare. Unlike other gastric surgeries, the stomach isn't opened, nor is any part of the stomach or intestine removed. However, there's a 5 percent failure rate because of balloon leakage, band erosion/migration, and deep infection. Also, some patients manage to continue "eating through" their band and, thus, don't lose weight. A sensible diet and exercise plan must be complementary to this surgery for optimal results.

Vertical Banded Gastroplasty Vertical banded gastroplasty (VBG) is one of the operations recognized by the National Institutes for Health for treatment of clinical obesity, the other being Roux-en-Y. VBG is a restrictive procedure that has no malabsorptive effect. The operation creates a small pouch at the top of the stomach with surgical staples and a polypropylene mesh band. The pouch initially can hold 1 ounce of food, but slowly expands to 2 to 4 ounces with time. The band regulates the size of the stoma and only lets a small bit of food through into the stomach, causing the patient to feel fuller faster and longer. The lower stomach can still digest food, just as with the adjustable gastric banding procedure, and there is no bypass of the small or large intestines.

The surgery is reversible, and the anatomy is left intact. Because there's no bypassing of the stomach or intestines, the patient is at lower risk for suffering nutritional deficiencies. However, someone who has this procedure must be motivated to stick to a strict diet afterward—a diet high in fat and sugar is a big no-no. If patients eat too much sugar, for example, it liquefies quickly in the pouch and moves rapidly through the stoma into the lower stomach, leaving the patient feeling hungry and wanting more food. Moreover, vomiting may be a problem if food is eaten too quickly or is not properly chewed.

VBG is a technically simple operation, and people might like it because nutritional deficiencies are rare. But the downside is that a third of patients who get this procedure tend to regain their weight. Therefore, it is recommended to highly motivated patients who can stick to a nutritionally sound diet.

Roux-en-Y Developed in the late 1960s, Roux-en-Y (RNY) has become the most common gastric bypass procedure due to its high success rates. It is also recognized by the NIH and is the procedure most preferred by bariatric surgeons because of its history of success and the research behind it. The Roux-en-Y procedure combines limiting food intake and bypassing part of the small intestine where absorption takes place. Because it solves two problems—appetite and absorption—greater weight loss can be achieved.

With the Roux-en-Y procedure, a portion of the stomach is sectioned off, creating a pouch that holds just 1 ounce of food or less. This causes a feeling of satiety after just a few bites. Then part of the small intestine is attached to the food pouch. Any food that passes through skips through the stomach and duodenum, the first part of the small intestine where food begins to be absorbed into the body.

you're not alone

When I graduated from high school, I weighed 450 pounds. After that, I just started gaining weight. When I got up to around 600 pounds, I tried to find help. I dieted. I saw doctors. Nothing worked.

In 1998, I looked into bariatric surgery. The doctor I saw told me I had to lose 200 pounds before he'd operate—back then, surgery wasn't as advanced as it is now. My choice was to get my jaw wired shut or lose weight on my own. I decided to go on a liquid diet, which I stuck to for 7 months and lost 90 pounds. It wasn't enough, so I gave up and went back to eating.

I was extremely depressed all the time. I didn't leave the house because I was so big. If I did, people would stare at me and make jokes. They know you're heavy, and they think you're deaf, too. During this time I was diagnosed with congestive heart failure, so I was in and out of the hospital a lot. If I left my house, it was in an ambulance.

In April 2001, I went into the hospital for congestive heart failure. My doctor told me the next time I checked into the hospital, I wouldn't be checking out. That's when I knew I had to do something. My mother came home with a paper from Ohio State University that said they were looking for applicants for bariatric surgery. I called for information and made an appointment. This doctor agreed to do the surgery on me. I weighed 745 pounds. I had to get the surgery because my option at that point was to die.

The surgery went okay—I had no complications. They used the Roux-en-Y gastric bypass procedure on me. In the first 30 days after I left the hospital, I lost 115 pounds. That was a real "Wow!"

Today I weigh 295 pounds (I'm 6'2"—a big guy) for a total weight loss of 450 pounds. I've had two plastic surgeries to remove a total of 50 pounds of excess skin from my body—I probably have another 50 pounds of excess skin left on me. I used to take 41 pills a day to treat diabetes, sleep apnea, my heart condition, and other health conditions affected by my weight—today, I take vitamin pills. That's it.

I travel now. I meet people. Best of all, I blend in. I don't stick out when I go to a restaurant or the mall. I have my first job, working in member services at ObesityHelp.com. I told myself that if I lost weight and made it through surgery, I'd help as many overweight people as I could. It has gone from me trying to get help to me helping other people. —*Kirk Thompson, 42, Ohio*

This procedure creates a "dumping syndrome" to control intake, especially of sweets. What happens with the "dumping syndrome" is that the lower part of the small intestine fills too quickly with undigested food from the stomach. The patient experiences symptoms of overeating including nausea, vomiting, and diarrhea. The feeling is unpleasant enough to discourage patients from overeating, so this negative side effect actually motivates patients to stay away from sweets. The other benefit of the Roux-en-Y procedure is that it's reversible in an emergency, although doctors urge patients to consider the surgery permanent. The downside includes staple line failure, ulcers, and narrowing and blockage of the stoma.

Biliopancreatic Diversion/Scopinaro Procedure Biliopancreatic diversion (BPD) is a less food-restrictive procedure than the Roux-en-Y procedure. The stomach holds 4 to 5 ounces, versus the single ounce of RNY. Like RNY, there's a significant malabsorptive component that helps with long-term weight loss. However, the patient needs to be monitored closely because of the risk of severe nutritional deficiencies. A benefit beyond malabsorption is that patients can eat larger quantities of food and still lose weight. However, there's a greater chance of chronic diarrhea, stomal ulcers, unpleasant smelling stools, and flatulence. Because of the malabsorptive component of the surgery, there's a high risk of nutritional deficiencies as well. Patients must be closely monitored by their physicians afterward.

Duodenal Switch The duodenal switch (DS) improves on the BPD procedure, which is why it's often called the BPD/DS. With DS, there's a significant malabsorptive component that helps in achieving long-term weight loss. Unlike BPD, this procedure keeps intact the pyloric valve, which regulates the release of the stomach's contents into the small intestine.

With the DS procedure, there's more normal absorption of many nutrients than with BPD, including calcium, iron, and vitamin B_{12}. The negative side effects of BPD are reduced or eliminated, as are the chances of developing a stomal ulcer. However, there's a greater chance for chronic diarrhea, a significant malabsorptive component, and more foul-smelling stools and flatus, but less than with BPD.

There's still a lot of debate and contention over the rapid increase of bariatric surgery procedures in this country. Some people, experts and laypeople alike, see bariatric surgery as an "easy way out" of obesity. The promise of an endless stream of patients has led some less-than-qualified doctors to pick up a scalpel and begin cutting, often with disastrous results.

However, for most people getting this surgery, the negatives far outweigh the positives. As Russell LaForte, M.D., points out, it is more dangerous for some of these patients to remain obese than it is for them to get the surgery with a highly trained bariatric surgeon. For these patients, it's often a choice between life and death.

Life after bariatric surgery isn't life on Easy Street. You can't expect to eat like you used to and still lose weight. Just like anyone else who loses weight and plans to keep it off, you've still got to change your behaviors and attitudes toward food and exercise.

> **WEB TALK:** Talk to people who've turned to bariatric surgery at:
> **ObesityHelp.com**

What You Can Do

If you've struggled your whole life with overweight and obesity and you think you've tried everything possible to lose weight, chances are, there's something new, something effective, something that will work for you. Don't give up hope. Researchers are working feverishly on new programs, behavior therapies, prescription drugs, gene studies, and surgeries to curb this worldwide health problem.

- ☐ Check out local colleges or universities, which may sponsor weight-loss programs staffed by trained professionals as an offshoot of their clinical nutrition or medical programs. Sometimes these programs are low cost—even free.

- ☐ If you have a medical condition such as diabetes, insulin resistance, heart disease, or hypertension, it's vitally important to work with your physicians on a weight-management plan that addresses these health conditions, too. Do not alter or vary your current diet plan without first consulting with them.

- ☐ Before you embark on a radical weight-loss plan (VLCD, prescription drug therapy, bariatric surgery), analyze your dieting history. Have you really tried everything to lose weight? What diet, exercise, and lifestyle changes could you make today that would make your life healthier, whether or not you pursue a radical solution to your weight?

- ☐ If you're thinking about bariatric surgery, consider attending a surgery seminar. Seminars, which are held by surgeons for a group of guests, allow you to gather information, ask questions, and get a feel for a doctor before you commit to an initial consultation. Check your local newspaper for announcements or call your local hospital.

- ☐ Some states cover the cost of obesity treatments for residents. Check with your state's health and human services and public health departments, as well as with your state's insurance commissioner.

- ☐ Second opinions count. Visit several bariatric practices before making any decisions.

Part 3

Working the Plan

You're excited. With the right diet along with the right mind-set, you're confident that this time you can lose weight. But before you begin, you should know some important things. Dieting is often easy to start, but without knowing where you're going, it's easy to get lost and discouraged. In these chapters, you learn how to plan the best outcome and how to cope with everything life will throw at you while you're dieting.

Before You Eat That Salad ...

Armed with information about all the kinds of diets out there, now the challenge is picking an eating plan you can live with.

Several years ago, I had lunch with a friend who was visiting the United States after living overseas for quite a while. I was stunned by her appearance. After having two children in close succession, she was amazingly slim. Her secret? She was following Atkins, which she embraced after a decade of low-fat dieting. I was intrigued. I began to research the diet, and within a few moments of looking at the food plan, the dismay set in. No bread? No pasta? And worst of all, the former vegetarian in me cried, "No fruits and veggies?" I did try the diet and lost 15 pounds. But my body and taste buds struggled with the increased animal proteins, and I felt deprived of my fruits and veggies. My physiology rebelled by developing frightfully bad breath and painful constipation.

Atkins, and low-carbing in general, simply didn't work for my mind-set, my food preferences, and my body. Many of my friends, however, have been able to embrace the low-carb lifestyle. They feel quite satisfied with the foods, and because many of them don't enjoy fruits and vegetables, the maintenance phase of the diet actually gets them to eat more complex carbs than they'd usually eat on their own.

Choose the Right Diet for *You*

One thing all the diet plans out there show us is that most diets work for *some* people *some* of the time. There simply isn't a diet that works for everyone *all* the time. This is good news for you, because it means there's probably a diet plan or two, or a combination of diet strategies, that will help you lose weight.

In a study published in the *Journal of the American Medical Association* (*JAMA*), researchers at Tufts–New England Medical Center in Boston assessed adherence rates and effectiveness of four popular diet plans in relation to weight loss and reduction of cardiac risk factors. The diets included Weight Watchers (calorie restriction), Atkins (carbohydrate restriction), the Zone (balance of carbohydrates, fats, and protein), and the Dean Ornish eating plan (fat restriction). Participating in the randomized trial were 160 overweight or obese adults ranging in age from 22 to 72 who had hypertension, high cholesterol, or high blood sugar levels. Forty randomized subjects were assigned to each diet, and for two months, the subjects had to follow the diet rigorously. After two months, they were allowed to choose their level of commitment to the assigned plan.

GET PSYCHED

"Leave your drugs in the chemist's pot if you can heal the patient with food."
–Hippocrates

The study demonstrated to researchers that the subjects who had the highest adherence levels to an assigned plan had statistically significant weight loss at one year. There was no statistical difference among the actual diets themselves, which is to say, for people who could commit to an eating plan, it didn't matter if they were eating saturated animal fats on Atkins or avoiding them on the Ornish plan. The *commitment* helped them lose their weight.

you're not alone

Six years ago, a friend wanted to lose a few pounds for her sister's wedding in June. So that March, we joined a weight-loss program I'd heard about at my church. But truly, I didn't hold out much hope I'd lose weight myself; it was more or less something I did to give her support.

I got a great head-start by catching the 24-hour stomach flu the day we began our new church-based eating plan. So after going a day without food, it was easier to tell when my now-shrunken stomach was full ... and being a bit weak from the illness, I wasn't inclined to crave much to eat in the first place. But after that, it truly boiled down to one meal at a time. Because there were no special foods, no charts, no calories/fat grams to count with my eating plan, I could live a normal life ... the willpower came in asking myself each time I reached for food, *Is your stomach growling? Or are you eating because you're bored? Sad? Think it's the best way to be sociable?* God gave us other outlets and tools for our emotional needs. Food is to fuel the body— not that it can't taste good, but it will never be love or acceptance, or any of the other things we try to make it be.

My husband thought it was wonderful, because by changing my eating behaviors instead of the menu, I didn't drag him into it by default, as in salads for dinner every night or refusing to eat in certain restaurants because they didn't fit my menu allowances. We saw our checks in restaurants drop as I started feeling satisfied with just the soup, or ordering the kiddie meals.

I make sure that when my stomach is growling, I put something in it rather than see how long I can hold on. That, to me, would be the beginning of a deeper problem. I also started out by believing I couldn't lose weight. I figured the extra pounds were just part of aging, and heaven knows, I wasn't willing to stick to a predetermined eating plan. So when the pounds started falling away, that became the motivation I needed to keep my portions small. I had no idea where it would bottom out ... and I was very curious to find out. After about a year, the scale stopped around 120 pounds.

Losing weight has to be about making yourself behave, not about making the food behave. The problem with most diets is that people can't or won't commit to eating that way for the rest of their lives. And without that, where are you when you stop the diet? Right back in the same habits that put on the poundage.

> Today I feel wonderful. Last year I felt light enough to start an exercise kick—now I walk 10,000 steps a day with the help of a treadmill parked smack in front of a big-screen television set! I'm back in a size 4, which is roughly where I was all through college and my early years of marriage, and I still get a little thrill when I try something on in the dressing room. Most folks have forgotten that I once carried the extra weight because I look like the person they've always known. —*Julie, 42, Indiana, permanently lost 60 pounds*

The researchers ended their article by suggesting doctors could improve their patients' success at weight loss by providing weight-loss options to better match the patients' food preferences, lifestyles, and cardiovascular risk factors. And because subjects in the study could not pick the diet they wanted to follow in the study, the researchers suspect adherence rates and clinical improvements would be even better if they had been allowed to choose according to their preferences.

What this seems to suggest is that what works is sticking to the diet, not the diet itself. So you have to ask yourself, *How do I pick a plan I'm more likely to stick with and not abandon after a few weeks?*

Food Preferences How many times have you picked up a diet book, all excited that this time you'll lose weight, and then feel your stomach drop as you start reading the list of "banned foods." No bread. No butter. No red meat. No carrots. No caffeine! And don't even think of having a bowl of ice cream ever again. Or you read the list of approved foods and nothing on it appeals to you. You notice half the meals don't include meat. Or if it's a low-carbohydrate plan, you wonder, where's your morning orange juice?

We all have foods we love. We all have foods we loathe. If you're considering a formal diet plan such as Atkins, or are deciding to embark on the vegetarian route, you've got to be realistic about how your food preferences are going to either support or doom your efforts.

It helps to have a clear picture of what your food preferences are. Start by writing a list of all the foods you enjoy—everything from the "bad stuff" (French bread, chocolate, and potato chips) to the "good stuff" (your favorite vegetables, beverages, and protein sources). Make the list as long and complete as possible. What foods on the list do you think would be hard to give up, even for the short term? What foods would you be willing to eat in moderation? For example, don't even try to talk me into giving up my morning coffee or afternoon tea. I love cheese, but I'd be willing to cut back on Brie to lose weight. And ice cream? I love it, but during times when I'm trying to drop a few pounds, I am fine with not eating it at all. But don't tell me I'll never be able to eat Ben & Jerry's again, because I'm going to resist it.

It's also a good idea to write down the foods you dislike. If vegetables make you turn green with disgust, write them down. Now's not the time to be hopeful your taste buds will change. If you're not a big meat-eater or hate fish, be honest with yourself. A weight-loss plan high in animal protein may be an exercise in futility for you.

If you're following a formal diet plan, weigh the diet's list of recommended and banned foods against your food lists. How do the lists compare? If you have a long list of grains and vegetables in your favorites column, and the diet you're considering restricts all carbohydrates, including complex carbs, you have to ask yourself how happy you're going to be on the diet. Many people find low-carb plans attractive because they emphasize foods they enjoy, such as red meat, eggs, and cream, and the diet takes the focus off vegetables and grains, the foods they don't really like. On the other hand, if pasta is one of your favorite foods, a strict low-carb plan may be difficult for you to follow. It may make more sense to figure out how you can incorporate a moderate amount of pasta into your diet.

With luck, you'll have a long list of healthy foods you enjoy. For example, my list includes strawberries, eggs, chicken, yogurt, salmon, tomatoes, asparagus, avocadoes, and shellfish. A plan that includes many of your healthy favorite foods will simply be easier for you to stick to over time. There will probably be some foods that must be limited if you're intent on losing weight, but the good news is that you can probably make some healthy substitutions. For example, I like eggs and could eat them every day, but eating eggs every day doesn't support my weight-maintenance goals. So when I make my Sunday morning omelet, I make it with one whole egg plus two egg whites. With a handful of chopped, fresh asparagus inside and a sprinkling of Parmesan cheese on top, this new and improved omelet satisfies my taste buds—as well as my scale.

GET PSYCHED

"Whatever diet you start now, you have to do forever. So pick something you can commit to for the rest of your life." —*Elena Ramirez, Ph.D., clinical assistant professor of psychology, University of Vermont, and director of UVM's Weight Control Program*

Lifestyle Before you choose a diet, you have to understand how your lifestyle will impact your weight-loss diet:

- Is this a plan you can stick to if you eat out frequently? If you have to travel for work or entertain clients, you want a plan that can work on the road and in restaurants.

- Is this a plan you can fit into your workday? If you work long hours and you choose a plan that requires a lot of food-prep work, how will you fit this into your schedule?

- Is this a plan that will work with your family's eating style? If you have to prepare two meals every night, are you going to get burned out in the kitchen? Or will you be able to eat the same foods as your family?

- Is this a plan you can stick to on vacations and holidays? You might be starting your diet when you don't have a lot going on in your life. But if you've got a cruise scheduled in a few months or you know holidays are a nonstop banquet for your family, it's better to understand up front what your options will be down the road.

- How much time do you want to spend preparing food? Some diet plans require a lot of attention to food prep and cooking. Let's get real: many of us want to spend as little time in the kitchen as possible. If shopping for special foods and preparing a week's worth of cut-up veggies makes your stomach sink, you'll want to think about choosing a plan that has less hands-on food prep.

- Examine your past dieting history and look where you had trouble. If you struggled with packing your own lunches every day, maybe it's better to develop a plan that allows you to pick healthy foods from your workplace cafeteria. On the other hand, if you can't resist the high-fat options at lunch, perhaps it's better to figure out how you can bring in your own meals. If you tend to overeat at client dinners, then maybe scheduling in time to eat a low-cal dinner before going out is a strategy you can use for your new eating plan.

Whatever diet you choose, you're going to have to make some changes and adjustments, and they won't feel natural or easy at first. Although you're busy at work, you may need to start carving out time to enjoy a quick lunch rather than skip a meal. But if you pick a diet plan that's overly complicated and time-consuming, you're probably going to go right back to your old eating habits—and gain even more weight.

Most of us are immensely busy. However, many successful dieters have overcome lifestyle obstacles such as busy jobs, non-stop travel, and family dining preferences to lose weight. The key? They went into their weight-loss program with their eyes open. For some of them, it simply meant giving their health and weight loss a higher priority on their to-do lists. If you're working 60- or 70-hour work weeks and not finding time to eat balanced meals and work out, consider this: taking a half-hour out of your day to walk or eat a balanced meal will actually help you perform better on the job. The walk will help you deal with stress. Do you really not have time to prepare foods? Can you trim 15 minutes off your TV time at night to make your lunch for the next day or wake up a bit earlier than usual to prepare food for the day? Do you always have to order the 20-ounce New York strip steak when you're out with clients, or could you substitute a salad topped with grilled lean meat?

GET PSYCHED

"I can eat, or I can eat what I *really* want. For me, it's all about making conscious choices about the foods I really want." *—Devin, Los Angeles, California*

Consider how your diet will fit into your schedule and the way you live your life. Make adjustments where necessary, but rather than squeeze your life into a diet plan, figure out how you can squeeze the diet plan into your life.

Working With Your M.D.

Whatever diet plan you choose, it's smart to visit your physician or any other medical specialists who care for you. Not only can they advise you on the diet plans you're considering, they can also perform medical tests to provide a benchmark for improvement or to possibly save your life. It's exciting to discover that after months of dieting, your cholesterol has dropped 20 points or your blood pressure is now in the normal range. These improved numbers can give you a boost of motivation during the midpoint of your diet. On the other hand, it's better to find out you have a health condition such as a blocked artery or high blood sugar before you go on a diet that could make the condition worse.

Another important reason to meet with your personal physician involves setting a goal weight. Your M.D. is going to be a good judge of your body type and health issues, and he or she may give you a goal weight that's more appropriate for your frame and health history than a table of numbers in a book can. Many dieters pick a weight goal for cosmetic reasons—they want to fit into a size 6 or they want to feel confident wearing a swimsuit. Mind you, there's nothing wrong with these goals if they are approached in a safe, healthy manner. But a physician might be able to give you a more reasonable and attainable intermediate weight goal. Your doctor is your cheerleader for your health, not just your looks and confidence levels. Research shows a 5 to 10 percent weight loss for many people brings tremendous health benefits, such as lower cholesterol levels, lower blood sugar, and a reduced risk of heart disease. There's nothing wrong with losing more, but an intermediate goal of health can be more realistic and valuable to you, especially if you have a lot of weight to lose.

Why does every diet book tell you to visit your personal physician before starting a weight-loss or exercise plan? Is this really necessary, especially if I'm in good health?

"A pre–diet/exercise checkup gives your physician a chance to screen for chronic medical problems that can be affected by your diet and exercise plans, such as coronary artery disease, hypertension, and diabetes. This physical allows your doctor to review your diet and exercise plans for their appropriateness to your individual health needs. For example, a person with arthritis may not do very well with an exercise plan that involves a lot of walking. With the age 40 and up crowd, screening for chronic medical conditions is more of a pertinent issue, but we see these problems in younger patients, too. Ideally, you should be getting a yearly physical, even if you're in good health."
–Caroline Rudnick, M.D., Ph.D., St. Louis University School of Medicine, family physician

In fact, research suggests, especially if you're obese, that your goal should be a modest reduction in weight, not necessarily getting down to your ideal weight. Given this advice, it's difficult for many dieters to figure out what a "modest amount of weight" means. Indeed, in a recent study conducted at the University of Pennsylvania, 60 obese women defined their weight-loss goals and assigned levels of happiness with the pounds lost. Rankings ranged from "dream weight" to "disappointed weight." When 47 percent of the women didn't even achieve their "disappointed weight goals," the study suggested that the medical profession needs to encourage even modest weight-loss outcomes.

Your Personal Weight-Loss Plan

As you're probably starting to figure out, weight loss occurs when certain behaviors and habits are repeated regularly, just as overweight and obesity occur when certain behaviors and habits are repeated regularly. Now it's time to decide what behaviors and habits you're going to adopt and which ones you're going to avoid.

These behaviors and habits are the answers to the "how" of your diet. If you want to reduce your body fat by 10 percent, you'll need to figure out how you're going to achieve this goal and adopt the right behaviors and habits to get you there. If you have a habit of skipping breakfast and eating lunch on the run, only to come home at night and gorge on anything at hand, you must figure out a better weight-loss strategy.

Before you start your weight-loss plan, you must get absolutely clear about what it is you do that keeps you from losing weight. Once identified, you need to figure out how you're going to change these behaviors for the betterment of your health and weight.

Planning Ahead If you've ever dieted and have been unsuccessful at losing weight permanently, you probably have some idea of what behaviors and habits led to your diet's failure. These behaviors and habits may include the following:

- Skipping meals and then overeating later
- Cheating on your diet one day and then figuring you've blown it, so you overeat on the following days until you give up the diet altogether
- Eating in front of the television
- Giving up on your diet when your weight plateaus or you experience weight gain for a few weeks
- Grocery shopping when you're hungry, which leads to filling your cart with unhealthful foods
- Eating mindlessly when you're bored, depressed, stressed, or angry
- Continuing to eat even when your stomach is full and you no longer feel hungry

157

Your food diary is a great place to start writing down all the behaviors and habits that haven't supported your weight loss in the past. After you have your habits in front of you in black and white, you can make plans about how you'll cope with them in the future.

For example, if you tend to sit in front of the television at night and mindlessly eat your way through your favorite programs, make a new rule that you'll only eat when you're sitting in a chair at the kitchen table. Or if the television snacking habit is too difficult for you to break right now, transition by agreeing with yourself only to eat low-cal treats such as air-popped popcorn or celery sticks. You can also create new habits for television-watching. Make a rule that whenever a commercial comes on, you will hop on your exercise bicycle and pedal for a few minutes. Get creative with your ideas—and write them down! You want to have many options at your disposal for the inevitable tough spots in your diet.

Robert Kushner, M.D., a professor of medicine at Northwestern University in Chicago, has studied dieters' eating, exercise, and coping patterns for 20 years. These patterns, he says, affect a person's ability to stick to a weight-loss program. For example, if you're the type who talks about losing weight but never seems to commit to a diet, Kushner would type you a "persistent procrastinator." A persistent procrastinator is going to have different issues from someone who diets, but because she sets such high expectations for herself, she never feels she's succeeding at weight loss (the "unrealistic achiever"). According to Kushner, only when you understand and work with your unique eating, exercise, and psychological coping patterns will you be able to stick with your weight-loss plan and, thus, lose pounds. (For more about Dr. Kushner's work and his three-dimensional weight-loss program, check out Appendix B.)

Every weight-loss plan I've been on recommends not skipping breakfast, but I'm just not hungry in the morning. How can I get around this?

"I endorse not skipping breakfast as well. Although we don't quite understand why it is important, most studies show that people who eat breakfast are more successful in managing their weight than those who skip that meal. With all new patients who skip breakfast, I first look at their nighttime eating habits because 'morning anorexia' is often due to excessive nighttime eating. 'Nighttime nibblers' get their fuel intake in the evening. Their bodies, which should be getting rest, spend the night digesting all that food. When these patients wake up, they're not feeling so hungry.

"I encourage patients to eat anything in the morning—a piece of fruit, some yogurt, a meal replacement bar—to get them into the habit of eating breakfast. It may take a while, but calorie intake can be shifted so the patient eventually starts feeling less ravenous at night and more hungry upon awakening."
—*Robert Kushner, M.D., medical director of the Wellness Institute at Northwestern Memorial Hospital and author of the* American Medical Association's Obesity Treatment Guide for Physicians

The Importance of Goals There are two types of goals with weight loss: your ultimate goals, a certain weight you want to hit and maintain for the rest of your life; and intermediate goals, which will help keep you motivated on your weight-loss journey.

Some dieters embark on a new weight-loss plan simply "to lose weight." Or they have a goal such as, *I should lose a few pounds around the middle* or *I'd like to lose 10 or 20 pounds*. But for many dieters, their ultimate weight-loss goal is nothing more than a vague hope that they can look like they did in college.

There's certainly nothing wrong with aiming for what you weighed in college as long as it's a healthy weight for your height and frame. But when you're dieting you have to develop weight-loss goals that are specific, achievable, and flexible. Telling yourself, *This time I'm going to lose 20 pounds* is better than *I'm going to lose weight*, because to make it really effective, you've got to make it a *specific* goal. Examples of specific goals include the following:

> *I will lose 20 pounds—an average of a pound a week— by May 1.*
>
> *I will bring my body-fat percentage to under 25 percent by December 1.*
>
> *I will get down to my target weight of 135 pounds by June 1.*

You see that each of these goals has specific weights, percentages, and dates attached to them, which means these are goals you can measure and quantify. In contrast, a goal of "losing weight" is hard to measure and quantify, which means it'll be difficult to monitor your progress.

Next is to be sure your goals are *achievable*. Aiming to lose 20 pounds in a month is just plain unreasonable, not to mention unsafe. You may have a goal of weighing what you did 10 years ago, and when you check weight charts, you find this is a reasonable goal for you. But if that means you've got to lose 100 pounds to hit this weight, it may be more achievable if you first create some intermediate weight-loss goals.

For example, my ideal weight is around 125 pounds for my height and frame. It's my ultimate goal weight. But I had to be honest with myself when I decided to lose weight once and for all—I'd been losing and gaining the same 10 pounds over the past 10 years and I knew I'd get discouraged trying to hit my ultimate weight goal. Instead, with the help of my physician, I set a more achievable, intermediate goal of getting my weight back down to the normal weight range for my height, which was also a weight I hadn't seen since before I got pregnant with my son. I found this goal much less daunting to go after, and within 6 weeks, I'd reached my goal. I felt great, I looked great, and I was more determined and inspired than ever to hit my ideal weight goal—which I eventually did, with the help of my intermediate goals.

The last key is *flexibility*. You may be thinking flexibility on a goal will give you wiggle room to cheat. *Au contraire.* Rigidity snuffs out more diets than flexibility. A flexible goal gives you room to accommodate for the inevitable roadblocks you'll encounter on your diet. For example, if you set a goal of working out on Mondays, Wednesdays, and Fridays and you start missing your Wednesday workout because of your son's soccer schedule, you may start feeling like you're failing on your diet. Rephrasing that goal to *I run for 30 minutes a day 3 times a week* gives you some options on the days you run, and it's a goal you're more likely to hit, especially if your schedule is unpredictable. Set yourself up for success, and you're more likely to meet your ultimate weight-loss goal.

> **WEB TALK:** Determine your body mass index (BMI) and find your healthy weight by visiting the National Institutes of Health's Aim for a Healthy Weight page at:
>
> **www.nhlbisupport.com/bmi/**

The next part of goal-setting is figuring out the "how" of losing your weight. Again, you'll want to pick strategies that are measurable, achievable, and flexible. The following table gives you some examples.

Phrasing Your Weight-Loss Strategies

Your Original Goal	A Better-Phrased Goal
I'm going to exercise more.	*I walk 30 minutes a day, 3 times a week.*
	I do weight training 3 days a week for a half-hour.
I'm going to eat less.	*I eat 1,800 calories a day; only 30 percent of those calories come from dietary fat.*
	I eat breakfast in the morning and eat lunch at my desk. I don't eat after 8 P.M.
I won't snack.	*I write in my food diary whenever I feel tempted to eat potato chips. If I have to have a snack, I eat salt-free pretzels.*
	I don't buy junk food at the grocery store. Instead, I keep my cupboards and refrigerator stocked with whole-grain crackers, low-fat spreads, and fruits and vegetables I love.

You'll notice the rephrased goals in the preceding table are written in the present tense, as if they're happening right this moment. Research shows that when goal-setters write down their goals as if they're already occurring, they have a better chance of achieving them because their brains behave as if they're already happening. That is, if you tell yourself with conviction you don't buy junk food when you're grocery shopping, chances are much better you'll stick healthful foods in your basket at the store than if you simply told yourself, *I'll try not to buy junk food.*

And yes, writing down your goals is important. Keep them where you can see them: taped to your bathroom mirror or tucked into the journal you write in every day. Even read them out loud to yourself, or repeat them as your mantra as you're driving to work. Eventually, your mind will help you do everything to make these goal statements a reality.

It's not enough to set goals, however. Goals must beget action ... persistent, consistent effort. When you've decided on an end goal and have plenty of goal strategies lined up, you have to make the time to follow through on achieving them. All your goals have to be broken down into actions you can take. For example, if your goal is to walk three times a week, you may need to create action items such as *Buy new walking shoes*, *Map out a walking route*, or *Walk on Monday, Wednesday, and Friday this week.*

Your Food and Exercise Diary One of the best tools to keep you focused on weight loss is a food and exercise diary. At its most basic level, a diary gives you a place to track the foods you eat each day. If you know you have to record every mouthful of food—that candy bar at 3 P.M., for example—a diary can give you an opportunity to think before you eat. Do you really want to ruin your good record with that junky snack? Wouldn't a more healthful snack look better in your journal—and on the scale?

You can capture all sorts of valuable information in a journal. If you struggle with emotional eating, write down how you feel whenever you want to reach for food. What time of day is it? What kind of emotional event occurred? What alternatives can you do besides eat? After a couple weeks of writing down your behaviors and feelings, you'll be able to see a pattern. Perhaps you reach for food when you're feeling stressed by your boss's unreasonable demands or you eat when you have nothing else to do. With this kind of self-knowledge at your fingertips, you can begin to work on the core issues behind your eating habits.

Journals are also a great place to track your goals, weight, victories, and athletic progress. When you're feeling down, you can pull out your journal. You'll have a written record of all the work you've done so far and can review all the great progress you've made and keep yourself motivated. Or if you find your weight loss isn't happening as fast as you'd like it to, a quick review of your journal may show you you've been eating more than you thought and exercising less.

Get creative with your journal. You can journal in a loose-leaf notebook, a bound journal you purchase at an art supply store, or even on your computer. Some people track their progress on their handheld computers. Here are some other ideas for journaling:

- Some commercial weight-loss programs offer online journaling for members. At WeightWatchers.com, for example, members can track daily food points on a personal web page as well as their daily exercise and weekly weight.

- You can download a daily food and exercise diary from the National Institutes of Health at www.nhlbi.nih. gov/ health/public/heart/obesity/lose_wt/diary.htm.

- There are literally hundreds of websites and computer programs for food and exercise journaling. Some of the best include Diet Power (www.dietpower.com), FitDay (www.fitday.com), NutriGenie (www.nutrigenie.com), Diet.com (www.diet.com), and DietOrganizer (www.dietorganizer.com).

- If a picture's worth more than a thousand words to you, use the power of your camera phone. Nutrax Corporation (www.nutrax.com) has developed a website that lets dieters upload photos of their meals into a picture-based food log.

- Many people have turned to blogging for everything from their hobbies to their families. If you don't mind sharing your diet with the world, you can blog your weight-loss journal. Check out www.blogger.com and www.movabletype.org for more information.

The Science of Nutrigenomics

As researchers unravel the mystery of the human genome, they are learning how to apply science and medicine to individuals, rather than to large groups of people. The pharmaceutical industry, for example, traditionally develops a drug to help treat a condition or disease found in thousands, perhaps millions, of people, regardless of genetic backgrounds. This one-size-fits-all kind of drug development results in some drugs that are not effective—or are even deadly—for certain individuals because of the way their particular body chemistries react to the drugs.

The new science of *pharmacogenomics* may help reduce adverse drug reactions. Scientists can study inherited variations in genes that dictate drug response, and they can explore the ways these variations influence a patient's good response, bad response, or lack of response to a drug.

In the same vein, researchers are beginning to apply what they're learning about genetic expression to the field of nutrition. This science is called *nutrigenomics,* and researchers hope to discover how genetic differences affect such things as nutrient absorption, metabolism, and excretion. Eventually, they hope to discover how to develop personalized diets and targeted

PsychSpeak

Nutrigenomics is the study of how nutrition affects health by altering the expression or structure of a particular genetic makeup. Similarly, **pharmacogenomics** is the study of how drugs affect a particular genetic makeup.

nutritional therapy for specific genotypes to prevent disease and maximize health and longevity. Perhaps this information will be used to influence recommended dietary allowance (RDA) guidelines established by the government for specific populations. Or eventually, when a baby is born, his or her genetic profile will be taken and a lifelong diet will be suggested for his or her specific profile to ensure optimal health and life.

The science of nutrigenomics is in its infancy, but already scientists and researchers are looking at ways the science can be applied to people today. A few companies are offering "customized diets" based on DNA analysis. You swab the inside of your cheek, send it to the company with a check, and they'll tell you what foods to consume and which ones to avoid based on your genetic profile.

But most scientists agree that nutrigenomics still has a lot of research ahead of it. It's still too soon to tell exactly how some nutrients interact with different body types. And there are ethical concerns. Some nutritionists question the importance of genetics with nutrition, because genetics just play one part in the obesity/ overweight puzzle. Unhealthy lifestyles and poor diets are still a problem for most people, not their genetic background. The allure of a nutrigenomic approach may make some marketers develop pills as quick fixes for people who don't want to make the necessary lifestyle and/or dietary changes that would do more for their overweight and obesity. Also, if genetic profiling becomes the norm, it opens up a Pandora's box of ethical questions: at some point, will health insurers be able to deny you health coverage if they find out you're not eating according to your genetic profile? Would you really want to know whether you have an increased risk for an illness such as Alzheimer's disease or cancer? And would you want your insurance company possibly knowing this information?

Even if there's a perfect diet for your genotype, almost every medical professional will agree: for now, you can do a lot to control your body's weight and health. All it takes is the right diet combined with strategies that work for your personality.

What You Can Do

Losing weight is rarely easy. If it was, far fewer of us would be looking for the magic weight-loss diet. But when you've prepared yourself prior to embarking on a plan, weight loss can go a lot easier for you than it has in the past.

WEB TALK: Learn about how nutrigenomics affects you as a consumer at:

www.mydna.com/genes/nutrigen/

☐ First, get a clean bill of health from your M.D. Work together on your weight-loss goals, and get some baseline tests you can compare with future tests.

☐ If you're thinking of following a formal diet plan, investigate the restrictions and demands it will put on you. Be honest with yourself up front about whether you'll be able to handle those restrictions and meet the demands.

☐ Talk to other people you know who've followed the diet plan you're considering. What did they enjoy about the plan? What was difficult for them?

☐ Try to figure out your biggest challenges before you start a diet. Chances are good these challenges will arise again. Decide ahead of time how you'll get through these challenges— and write down your strategies so you can see them when you need them!

☐ Consider modifying a formal diet plan to your own tastes. For example, if you'd really like to try a low-carbohydrate plan but the thought of giving up fruit for 4 weeks is unappealing, don't give up the fruit. Having a cup of berries in the morning and an apple in the afternoon is not what's making you gain weight.

☐ Set realistic, achievable, and flexible goals—and don't forget to set some intermediate goals, especially if you've got a lot of weight to lose. Celebrate losing your first 25 pounds or being able to run a mile without stopping.

The Role of Exercise

When you're overweight, exercise is often the last thing you want to do. Exercise is hard work. It can be inconvenient, and sometimes it's not fun, especially when you haven't done it in a while. On top of that, when you're overweight you may have a lot of negative associations with exercise. You were the "fat kid" who was always picked last for sports. You resist exercise because you worry about how your thighs will look in jogging pants. So you put off exercise. You think, *When I lose more weight and look better, I'll start exercising.*

But let's look at the flip side. Exercise *makes* you look better. It doesn't have to be hard work. It can turn into an activity you look forward to—even crave. It can actually be *fun*. And although you may have some negative associations about exercise, I'm here to assure you that millions of overweight and formerly overweight people have learned to overcome them—and so can you. I talked to dozens of former exercise evaders who now can't go a day without moving. In fact, I was one of them. I was *always* picked last for sports when I was younger, and I avoided the gym for years because I hated exercising in public. Today, I'm training for my first sprint distance triathlon. That's a half-mile swim, a 12-mile bike ride, and a 3.1-mile run in one day, one event right after the other, in front of hundreds of people. And I'm 40. So I understand where you are, because I've been there.

The best news of all about exercise: it will actually *help* you lose weight, easier than almost anything else you can do. It's the magic pill you've been looking for, and it works. Not only will you lose weight faster, but nearly every other aspect of your life will improve—from your looks and your self-confidence to your relationships and moods.

Our Innate Drive to Move

It seems almost simplistic to say, but human beings are compelled to move. Hundreds of thousands of years ago, sitting around all day would have been dangerous to our species, not just our health. We'd be a lot lower on the food chain today if *Homo sapiens* treated movement as an option rather than a necessity. They wouldn't have eaten, and they would have *been* eaten.

Lucky for our ancestors (as well as us), they had brains and muscles. They used their intelligence to help them move faster and more efficiently. They learned how to outwit predators, some of whom were a lot stronger. They moved to find more hospitable climates for their tribes and families. They followed animal herds and used speed and strength, as well as cunning, to feed their kin. It was a lot of hard work, but we can see our ancient ancestors also enjoyed moving for the sheer enjoyment of it. Dance, after all, has its roots in prehistory.

Our ancestors developed tools such as traps, nets, and guns so they wouldn't have to chase after food. They trained animals to perform heavy labor so they didn't have to. But even in the past 400 or 500 years, people haven't been able to stop moving. Life may have gotten a little easier, but it was still hard work. Interestingly, our more recent ancestors, who definitely had more physical daily lives than we do, had the time and energy to develop sports such as Olympian events, tennis, and baseball.

In the twentieth century, when we had more time than ever for these downtime activities, something happened. We stopped moving. And because we weren't moving all that much during the workday, we set ourselves up for a health crisis.

Children and Movement Have you ever watched young children at play and caught yourself saying, "I wish I could bottle up all that energy and use it myself?" Observe a group of preschoolers sitting around in a circle. They can't sit still. They fidget. They wiggle. Soon, they can't sit still any longer. They start edging away from the circle to explore something that's caught their attention. They start stretching, hopping around. Next thing you know, they're off and running.

Then children head off to school, where they spend increasing amounts of time sitting down. As they get pulled into the educational system, less time is available for play and physical activity. Some children get involved with organized sports and dance. A great number don't. Alarmingly, many schools are cutting back on physical education and organized sports programs to reduce budgets. As a result, many children may learn the message that fitness is less important than reading, writing, and arithmetic. It's something optional, a line item that can be cut with little consequence to the big picture.

It's no wonder research shows that more children are spending less time participating in physical activities on their own. The Centers for Disease Control report that more than one third of children in grades 9 through 12 don't participate in any vigorous physical activity. Forty-three percent of children in these grades watch television more than 2 hours a day. As children enter adolescence, their physical activity levels drop dramatically. Those levels are even more dramatic with adolescent females, who are significantly less likely than adolescent boys to participate in vigorous physical activity.

So let's get back to those preschoolers and your wistful thoughts about their energy. Unfortunately, science hasn't yet figured out a way to bottle youth—but you most certainly can get a measure of that joyful enthusiasm on your own, no matter your age, weight, sex, lifestyle, or health.

The secret? Like those kids, you've got to get up and get moving.

Why the Drive Gets Blocked As we enter adulthood, we gain more responsibilities. There's college or work. We buy homes. We start families. We do something that's practically part of the American Dream. It's called "settling down," and you can read into that literally and figuratively.

PsychSpeak

Someone who is **sedentary** engages in no physical activity during leisure time—no exercise, sports, or hobbies requiring movement.

The statistics about activity levels of American adults are pretty dismal. Data collected from a 1997 through 1998 National Center for Health Statistics survey showed that nearly 40 percent of adults participated in no leisure-time physical activity. Beyond eating, sleeping, and performing basic functions necessary to sustain life, these people are essentially *sedentary*.

Physical activity levels *do* tend to decrease as people age. In addition, our metabolisms slow down. We tire more easily. We become more vulnerable to illness and injury. But plenty of evidence shows even the oldest people in our society can and do benefit from regular exercise. However, the same data from the National Center for Health Statistics showed that one third of people over the age of 65 lead sedentary lifestyles, and older women are more likely to be sedentary than older men.

As you can see, the Great American Slowdown isn't occurring because of biology. It's happening when we're children, when we have energy reserves to spare. By the time many of us enter adulthood, we get out of breath walking to the dinner table. If we can't blame biology, what else is to blame?

First, technology. Few people will argue that technology has made our lives more difficult, but it certainly has reduced the number of activities we do that burn calories. Our ancestors, by necessity, spent their lives performing backbreaking labor—everything from hunting for food to cultivating land. They didn't *need* a formal exercise plan—they burned an extraordinary number of calories each day just trying to survive.

Today, we don't walk—we drive. Indeed, many communities have fewer sidewalks than they did 20 years ago. We don't have to spend months crossing the Rockies in a covered wagon—we fly over those mountains in a plane. We don't cut our lawns with hand threshers. We have mowers, and many of us even do lawn mowing while we're sitting. We have televisions and computers, video games, and iPods. We are bombarded with a constant stream of information and data, so much so that we feel we need a break. And

WEB TALK: Find out what percent of the population in your city, state, or nation is physically active at: www.cdc.gov/nccdphp/dnpa/physical/stats/us_physical_activity/index.htm

how do many of us take this break? We sit down with a bowl of ice cream in front of the television. We put up our feet, and we try to relax.

The second thing to blame may be genetics. In a fascinating study conducted by James Levine, M.D., a Mayo Clinic endocrinologist, 10 obese subjects and 10 lean subjects were outfitted with customized, data-logging undergarments that monitored body postures and movements through sensors every half-second over 10 days. The data show that the difference between the lean and the obese could be accounted for by one factor—NEAT, or nonexercise activity thermogenesis—a fancy way of saying normal, everyday activities. The obese subjects sat, on average, 150 minutes more per day than their leaner counterparts, leading them to burn 350 fewer calories per day. Even when obese patients lost weight during the study, they still sat more than the lean subjects, and when the lean subjects gained weight, they didn't sit more. Such findings suggest that NEAT is fixed.

"Our patients have told us for years that they have low metabolism," Levine said in the journal *Science,* which published the results of the study in 2005, "and as caregivers, we have never quite understood what that means—until today. Our study shows that the calories that people burn in their everyday activities— their NEAT—are far, far more important in obesity than we previously imagined." Levine sums it up by asking physicians to encourage their patients to boost their NEAT. All it takes is standing instead of sitting to perform many simple tasks.

And yes, aging is partially responsible for why we slow down. Research shows that humans lose 10 percent of lean body mass every decade after the age of 18. When we lose muscle mass, metabolism slows. We tire more easily and become more vulnerable to illness and injury. But research also demonstrates that regular exercise can slow the aging process considerably. Older people who exercise can avoid many of the age-related conditions affecting their peers. Although the aging process is something none of us can avoid, we can certainly embrace it in better physical condition.

The Physiological Benefits of Exercise

When we engage in regular exercise over an extended period of time, it causes all our systems to perform better. Not only do we lose fat and gain muscle, but our hearts get stronger as well. Our bodies learn to process oxygen more efficiently, which boosts metabolism. We reduce our risk of developing life-threatening diseases. Our bones stay strong. We look better. We live longer. We live *better*. What's not to love?

Lisa Dorfman, R.D., is a sports nutritionist and competitive runner and triathloner who works with athletes in Miami, Florida. She says exercise physically improves our bodies in three phases.

The first phase involves building cardiovascular strength. When we're building cardio strength through *aerobic exercise,* we're teaching our bodies how to burn fat. Exercise changes the way our bodies use calories. Our bodies eventually learn how to efficiently burn energy off our fat stores during exercise, which assists weight loss.

In the second phase, you build muscle mass through *strength training*. When you

PsychSpeak

There are three types of exercise. **Aerobic exercise** (also called cardiovascular conditioning) builds heart strength and improves the respiratory system. Examples of aerobic exercise include fitness walking, running, and swimming. **Strength training** builds muscle mass and endurance; pumping iron or walking with hand weights are examples. Last is **stretching**, which keeps muscles nimble and flexible. Activities such as yoga, Pilates, and gentle stretching help with maintaining flexibility. An effective fitness plan includes all three types of exercise.

have more muscle mass, your body burns more energy. That means you burn fat while you're sleeping, eating, or watching TV. Sounds too good to be true? Here's the reason: your body requires 3 calories to maintain 1 pound of fat. It requires anywhere from 35 to 50 calories to maintain 1 pound of muscle. Do the math. You may have a friend who has 10 pounds on you, eats like a horse, and never gains weight, but if she has a *body fat percentage* of 22 and yours is 40 percent, she's burning off more calories than you are each hour. It's also a reason why men tend to lose weight easier than women; men typically have more muscle mass than women. *Stretching* is also important for muscles; stretching exercises keep your muscles loose and flexible.

The third phase is about maintenance. It's the exercise you do to keep your body in peak physical condition. Dorfman says it's important to keep this exercise purposeful and fun. At this point in the game, some days you don't have time to exercise or you don't feel like it, but you do it anyway, just as you brush your teeth twice a day. You may even be addicted to it. And it has other benefits as well. Says Dorfman, "On the days I'm tired, I use that time to pray, to be spiritual, to plan my day, and strategize. Exercise isn't for the sole purpose of exercise—it helps me to master other areas of my life."

PsychSpeak

Knowing and understanding your **body fat percentage** is a valuable weight-loss tool. When you know how much of your body is fat, you can more accurately assess your weight and fitness levels. Muscle weighs more than fat, so many dieters who exercise get discouraged when they gain. However, if they're tracking their body fat percentage, they'll often find a gain of muscle and loss of fat. More muscle means more fat-burning. Some home scales determine body fat, or you can get it tested at a gym or with a health professional.

Improved Cardiovascular Function

The benefits of regular exercise to your heart are numerous. Study after study shows people who exercise regularly suffer less heart disease and reduce risk factors for heart attacks than those people who don't move. Exercise prevents the deposits of cholesterol in blood vessels that lead not only to atherosclerosis but to high blood pressure.

Your heart is a muscle, just like the muscles in your thighs or arms. The only way it can get stronger is when it moves more. And the only way you can get it to move is by making it work— or beat—harder. When your heart is strong, it can pump blood more efficiently throughout your body. It also beats fewer times per minute, which saves wear and tear on the muscle. It can actually beat more powerfully with less effort than an unfit heart.

The American Heart Association urges everyone to exercise for heart health. Even if you're totally inactive, doing something is better than doing nothing. Its studies show that moderate exercise offers protection to the heart. In fact, moderate exercise obtained through an activity such as walking may be better for your heart than more vigorous exercise such as running. The key is doing something, anything, to get your heart beating faster.

One thing new exercisers complain about is a feeling their hearts are going crazy when they exercise. Some describe it as feeling like their hearts are slamming against their ribs. Others just feel uncomfortable and nauseated. You should always visit your doctor before starting an exercise program so your heart's health can be evaluated. It's absolutely critical to schedule

WEB TALK: The American Heart Association's online fitness center helps you plan an exercise program for heart health at:

www.justmove.org

this visit if you have other health problems besides overweight and obesity.

Again, your heart is a muscle. You wouldn't expect to bench press 200 pounds if you've never lifted weights, but many new exercisers force their hearts to perform similar feats of strength, with disappointing results. The key to building cardiovascular strength is training this muscle gently and slowly. If it exhausts you today to walk around the block, begin by walking around the perimeter of your house. Do it again tomorrow, and the day after that. When you feel comfortable with one lap, add a second lap. Then a third. Eventually your heart will strengthen so you can start walking around the block.

PsychSpeak

Your **target heart rate** is the number of beats per minute (BPM) at which your heart should work during exercise. It is expressed as a range which is determined by age—younger people have a higher target heart rate than older people. The American Heart Association recommends that you work out at a range between 50 and 75 percent of your maximum heart rate while performing aerobic exercise.

Another tool to building cardiovascular strength is exercising within your *target heart rate*. You can determine if your heartbeat is falling within this range via low-tech means such as taking your pulse, or via high-tech equipment such as with a heart monitor. To take your pulse manually, touch your fingers to your pulse point on the opposite wrist or gently touch the pulse point on your neck. Count your heartbeat for 6 seconds, and multiply it by 10 to get your heart rate.

A fitness professional can work with you to be sure you're exercising within your range.

Target Heart Rates Based on Age

Age	Target HR Zone (50% to 75%)	Average Max HR (100%)
20	100 to 150 BPM	200 BPM
25	98 to 146 BPM	195 BPM
30	95 to 142 BPM	190 BPM
35	93 to 138 BPM	185 BPM
40	90 to 135 BPM	180 BPM
45	88 to 131 BPM	175 BPM
50	85 to 127 BPM	170 BPM
55	83 to 123 BPM	165 BPM
60	80 to 120 BPM	160 BPM
65	78 to 116 BPM	155 BPM
70	75 to 113 BPM	150 BPM

Metabolic Benefits What's really exciting about exercise is how it affects your metabolism, or the rate you burn energy. The bottom line is that exercise builds muscle mass and burns off excess fat, which improves your metabolic rate.

Metabolism tends to slow as we age. As we approach middle age, we start to lose muscle mass and replace—or increase—that weight with fat. And as I've discussed earlier, the body needs less energy to maintain a pound of fat than it does a pound of muscle. This is why strength training, which builds muscle, is so beneficial for metabolism. People who remain physically active

PsychSpeak

Your **maximum heart rate** is about 220 minus your age. For example, a 30-year-old's maximum heart rate would be 220 – 30 = 190 BPM. Your target heart rate can be determined by multiplying that number by 50 and 75 percent.

throughout their lives tend to stave off a slowing metabolism. In fact, many men and women over 40 have faster metabolisms now than they did when they were young, for the simple fact they're more physically fit than they were at 20.

Cancer Prevention The research is promising on how exercise reduces the risk of developing cancer. Even when risk factors for a certain type of cancer are high, such as a genetic component, exercise can help reduce the chance of developing the disease.

The effect of exercise on breast cancer risk is extremely promising. Some risk factors for the disease are not easily changed, such as having a mother or sister who had the disease, or delaying or forgoing childbirth. Research shows, however, that engaging in a vigorous exercise program reduces a woman's risk of developing breast cancer by 30 percent.

There's a strong link between people with inactive lifestyles and higher rates of colon cancer. The American Cancer Society says that even a moderate program of exercise can reduce risk.

Regular exercise, along with weight reduction, may also reduce the risk of developing endometrial cancer, kidney cancer, oral and esophageal cancers, and pancreatic cancer.

Increased Bone Density Loss of bone density is a problem for people when they're aging. Postmenopausal women are especially vulnerable. One of the best ways to prevent bone density loss is exercise, especially weight-bearing or resistance exercises. Any time you make your bones and muscles work against gravity, you're engaging in weight-bearing exercise; examples include walking and stair climbing. Resistance exercise develops muscle mass and strengthens bones; examples of this type of exercise are lifting weights and using resistance bands. Just as your muscles grow stronger with exercise, so do your bones, which actually become denser with use. Moreover, stronger muscles help you become more coordinated and less likely to fall and injure bones.

Studies prove that exercise delivers big benefits to your bones. In a recent German study, postmenopausal women with signs of bone density loss were instructed to exercise four times per week—two times in a group session, and two times at home. Five months into the study, the researchers added jumping exercises to stimulate the bones by promoting muscle movement. The results were promising. In subjects who stuck with the program for 26 months, researchers noted less bone loss in the spine and hip, less back pain, and more physical strength, among other benefits.

Improved Muscle Tone One of the aesthetic benefits of exercise, when combined with weight loss, is how it makes you look. Dieters who don't exercise often find themselves looking quite flabby after they've lost weight. If you build muscle mass while losing weight, your skin has a chance to slowly adapt to the new shape of your body. Especially when you're losing weight rapidly and not exercising, your skin has no muscles to mold to. So it bags and sags around your body, causing your body to look years older than it really is.

When your muscles are taut and toned, your clothes fit better and you feel more comfortable in them. You can start wearing clothes you may have avoided in the past: sleeveless tops, shorts, skirts. This, in turn, makes you feel even better about yourself.

Good muscle tone protects you from injury. If you've been having back problems, for example, strengthening the muscles that support your torso can reduce, even eliminate pain. When you combine exercise with weight loss, the results can be even more dramatic. You literally take a weight off your back.

Hormonal Changes Many people place the blame for weight problems on their *hormones,* and they're partially right. Hormones do influence weight gain. However, hormones are also responsible for helping us lose weight, and as research shows, hormones can be manipulated through diet and exercise.

Insulin is one such hormone that can be regulated through exercise. Insulin is secreted by the pancreas, and it helps your body process blood glucose (blood sugar). When this process works, glucose moves from the blood stream into the cells, providing energy.

However, many people struggling with overweight or obesity have problems with insulin regulation. They may be insulin-resistant, which means normal amounts of insulin don't work, so the body produces even more insulin to compensate. Their problem is not a lack of insulin, but a loss of sensitivity to it. In some people, eventually even the excess insulin has no effect on blood glucose, so glucose builds up in the bloodstream, resulting in type 2 diabetes.

PsychSpeak

Hormones are chemical substances produced throughout the human body, which are then carried through the bloodstream to direct changes in other parts of the body. Hormones are responsible for directing everything from the development of sex characteristics to mood regulation.

you're not alone

When I was in college, I started gaining weight. I was on a fencing team for the first 2 years, so I got some exercise, but during my last 2 years I didn't do any exercise at all. On top of that, I didn't eat well—I didn't know about calories or what foods were best for me.

After college, I moved to New York City. Then my priority was finding a job and a place to live, not finding a gym or losing weight—it wasn't part of my thinking. So I continued to gain weight.

I got up to about 150 pounds—I'm not sure how much exactly, because I didn't weigh myself a lot—but I went to see a doctor. When she saw my weight she told me I had to do something, and that was depressing. Someone finally noticed I was getting heavy. I thought, *I'm young, I deserve to eat what I want,* so I didn't listen to her.

The turning point for me came in August 1999 when I signed up for a swing dance class. There were all these mirrors around the room, and I couldn't hide: I was definitely not looking like me. The other turning point was when I had to start wearing a size 14. I'm 5'2". I started educating myself about calories and how many I needed each day to stay healthy and lose weight. Then I made some small changes, like substituting Diet Coke for Coke, cutting out fried foods, and eating more vegetables. I also joined a gym and started working out.

By the time December rolled around, I'd lost 15 pounds. That's when I met Marc, my boyfriend. He's super athletic, so I found myself doing more athletic activities, like running in the park instead of on the treadmill at the gym. That's when my body shape really changed.

One day I was talking to a friend who wanted to do a triathlon. At that point, I was reasonably fit. It was scary-exciting to consider. I thought, *I don't know if I can do this, but I have to try.* Plus, it was the one thing Marc hadn't done, nor had my athletic brother, and that was appealing. I knew I would enjoy the accomplishment, but what I didn't expect was that I'd enjoy the actual event, which I completed in the summer of 2004—it was so much fun. And the training was great, too. It was never boring—one day I would run, the next day I'd swim or bike. Now I'm hooked.

I used to hate running—it was so hard, so painful. My heart would pound, it was hard to breathe, and I hurt all over. But the more I did it, the easier it got. Today I actually look forward to it—all those endorphins! *—Sarah S., 28, New York City*

Because one benefit of exercise is that it helps burn off fat, this can help people who are insulin-resistant tremendously. These people tend to collect weight around their midsection, which has a big impact on their blood sugar control. A lean body mass also improves glucose metabolism. Consequently, an exercise program that develops muscle mass and reduces fat improves insulin resistance.

The Psychological Benefits of Exercise

Hormones are also responsible for one of the most pleasing side effects of exercise: mood control. In fact, many avid exercisers cite a psychological need rather than a physical need to exercise. Sure, they love the way their bodies look and they appreciate the effects exercise has on their metabolisms, but what gets them off and running is the way exercise makes them feel inside their own heads.

Fight Stress and Depression If you've been inactive all your life, or you're simply at the point where you don't enjoy exercise, it's hard to believe that someday exercise will begin to make you feel better. You'll actually look forward to it because of the positive chemical reactions it stimulates in your brain. This "high" is the same kind of "high" you get by eating chocolate or making love!

People who exercise regularly often report a feeling of euphoria during and after exercise, sometimes up to 12 hours after the activity has ended. This is because during prolonged exercise, the brain releases neurotransmitters called endorphins, which have chemical qualities similar to opiate drugs. Scientists aren't sure why the body responds to exercise this way. A simple explanation is that the nervous system responds to certain kinds of stress by releasing these pain-killing neurotransmitters ... and exercise happens to be one of those "stresses." It is no wonder that so many people become addicted to exercise.

Exercise helps fight depression and anxiety. Many medical professionals recommend physical exercise for patients suffering from these psychological conditions. Sometimes, exercise alone alleviates symptoms of mild depression and anxiety. In a study published in the journal *Professional Psychology: Research and Practice*, researchers discovered that subjects diagnosed with clinical depression were significantly less depressed after 5 weeks of walking, running, or doing strength-training exercises 3 times a week for 20 to 60 minutes. When subjects kept up with their workouts, the positive effects of exercise lasted until the study's end.

Moreover, relieving stress through exercise is good for your heart. It gives your body a release of the chemicals that cause your body's nerve centers to go into overdrive. When you're stressed, your heart beats faster, but it's not because you're moving more. It's because your body is pumping out adrenaline, a hormone that prepares your body for intense activity, particularly the fight-or-flight reaction. You get a feeling of "burnout" when your body produces too many stress hormones. A better way to get your heart beating— and to burn off stress—is through exercise.

GET PSYCHED

"Not only is exercise a viable treatment option for mild to moderate depression, it is four to five times more cost-effective than traditional forms of psychotherapy." *—Gregg Tkachuk, Ph.D. candidate in clinical psychology at the University of Manitoba in Canada, quoted in* Psychology Today, November/ December 1999

Look Better, Feel Better When you get a new hairstyle that flatters your face, every time you catch a glimpse of yourself in a mirror, you might think, "Hey, I look pretty good!" and you stand a little taller. Or you lose a bit of weight and fit into a favorite pair of jeans you'd outgrown. Or you remember the way you felt on your wedding day. You look good, so you feel good. Friends, even strangers, notice and comment. You become more confident, optimistic, ready to tackle the world. And because you feel great, life at those moments is a lot easier to handle.

I feel self-conscious about exercising. How can I get over the fear that people are staring at me?

"This is more of a body issue problem, and it's very common. It's probably not the only thing overweight people avoid, and avoidance and feeling bad just make people generally eat more. If there's an underlying body image issue going on, I always refer people to therapy for that. Exposure therapy, which is doing something you're anxious about despite anxiety and doing it until you feel less anxious, is the answer here.

"In the short term, however, dieters need to exercise. I suggest they have an in-home exercise option, such as exercise tapes, a treadmill, or a stationary bike. This doesn't mean they should avoid exercising in front of others and keep feeling they need to hide in their homes. This is why the behavioral therapy is important." *—Elena M. Ramirez, Ph.D., licensed psychologist-doctorate and director of the University of Vermont's Weight Control Program*

It's a psychological truth—when you like the way your body looks, you feel better about yourself. Certainly you've noticed the opposite is true ... when you're out of shape, not eating well, and you're putting on the pounds, you tend not to like the reflection in the mirror. You avoid buying clothes because nothing fits right, or the clothes show how big you've become. If you're in a relationship, you start avoiding sex because you're ashamed of the way your body looks to your partner. And if you're seeking a relationship, you feel less confident about your ability to attract a partner. In all aspects of your life, you feel anxious or depressed. And because you feel anxious and depressed, you crawl even further into your shell.

While interviewing formerly overweight and obese people for this book, the one thing that struck me was how ashamed they were of their bodies. Many of them avoided exercise for years because they were afraid people would stare at them, or worse, laugh. Some of them hid from the world in their homes, eating more, exercising less and less, until they were in grave danger of losing their health and possibly their lives.

But after they shed pounds and started to move, they began to notice how good—really good—their bodies were looking. And because they felt good about the way they looked, they were even more inspired to exercise. The aspects of their lives they felt insecure about in the past—everything from work and leisure activities, to relationships and their sex lives—suddenly changed when they started looking better. Says Kelly, a sales executive from Detroit, "Looking good and feeling good has reenergized my marriage and sex life. I just *feel* more sexual."

These people lost the weight and managed to work through the issues they had about exercise. They started off slow— many walked, others joined gyms—but they got out there. As the weight dropped away and their muscles got used to the exercise, they started to exercise more and worry less about what people thought of them.

GET PSYCHED

"I've always loved sleeveless shirts, but I avoided wearing them when I was heavy. When I lost weight and started getting in shape, the first thing I did was buy a bunch of sleeveless outfits to show off my toned arms."
—*Sarah S., New York, New York*

More Energy, More Brainpower It seems almost counterintuitive that by expending more energy you gather more energy. It's a law of physics: a body in motion tends to stay in motion; a body at rest tends to stay at rest. Energy begets more energy. But haven't you noticed yourself that on a purely unscientific level, the most energetic, lively people you know tend to move around a lot more than people who aren't as peppy?

We've established that regular exercise can affect hormone levels in the body such as insulin. Some researchers believe that exercise may also lower levels of the hormones that overstimulate the nervous system, including adrenaline and cortisol, while improving the levels of melatonin, a hormone produced in the brain that helps us sleep at night. When we get enough restful sleep, we wake up more energized and refreshed. But when our bodies become overloaded with stress hormones, we don't sleep as well. Our energy reserves deplete, and we drag ourselves through the day.

Exercise may also improve our ability to think and solve problems. Our brains definitely benefit from increased oxygen levels. Researchers are intrigued by the idea that brain function can be improved through exercise. In a study conducted by the Beckman Institute and Neuroscience Center in Illinois, researchers found that cardiovascular-fit subjects had better functioning in the attention network of their brains during certain cognitive tasks compared to subjects who were not as fit or who didn't exercise at all.

WEB TALK: Search for individual and group sports and activities by zip code at:

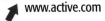 www.active.com

Choosing the Right Exercise Plan for You

Choosing an exercise plan is a little like choosing a diet plan: you have to choose something you have a chance of following over the long term. For example, if you travel a lot for work, it might not make sense to sign up for a series of aerobics classes, because you may not be able to attend them regularly. Find an activity that fits into the life you have today. After exercising starts to become part of your life, you can look for ways to schedule your life around exercise!

When Lisa Dorfman, R.D., a Miami-based sports nutritionist, begins working with new clients, she asks them to answer her five W's and one H before they choose an exercise plan:

- **Who** are you exercising with? If you're exercising on your own, will you feel isolated?

- **What** do you need? Make a list of any special equipment: clothes, running shoes. Are you ready to make a financial commitment for these items?

- **Where** do you exercise? If you travel a lot, for example, you might want to pick an exercise program you can do on the road.

- **Why** are you exercising? Is it for weight loss? What are your other exercise goals?

- **When** are you going to exercise? Do you have to make an appointment for your workout? Can you only work out at night?

- **How** are you going to exercise? Will you need a coach or a fitness instructor? Can you read a book or magazines to get the knowledge you need?

If you haven't exercised in a while, pick an exercise you know you can do right now. Walking, says Dorfman, is one of the best ways to exercise, because there's virtually no learning curve. "You can walk your dog, walk with your kids, a friend, and it makes exercise fun," she says. "You can walk to work or to school. The key is to make exercise purposeful. Not only will you enjoy it, but you'll begin to lose weight."

Making Exercise a Habit

According to the International Health, Racquet, and Sportsclub Association, more people join health clubs in January than in any other month. In fact, one third of all membership sales are made in the first three months of the year, when people tend to be gung-ho about getting in shape.

The new members show up at the gym every day. They pump weights the first day, then show up the next, sore and tired, to do a half-hour on an elliptical trainer. After a couple weeks of this madness, they start slacking off on the gym visits. Eventually, they stop going at all. Why? It's not fun. Working out hurts, and they're not seeing results. The fact that they're still paying off a pricey membership contract adds yet another layer of guilt.

There's nothing wrong with getting excited about an exercise plan. I encourage you to get *very* excited—exercise will do wonders for your body as well as your mind! However, I urge you to ditch the all-or-nothing approach to exercise. It's far better to go with a slow-and-steady approach.

When you take the slow-and-steady approach, you're able to train yourself to look forward to exercise. If you jump on a treadmill and try to push your body to do more than it can, it will resist you. You'll spend the whole session gasping for air and feeling miserable. The next day you'll probably feel sore and tired. It's no wonder resistance sets in the next time you approach the treadmill—your brain is screaming, *This isn't fun!*

WEB TALK: Track your exercise progress for free at: www.fitday.com

However, a slow-and-steady approach gives your body time to adjust to the new demands you're putting on it. So if you've decided to walk on a treadmill, figure out what you can do *today*. It may be 5 minutes. It may be 1 minute. It doesn't matter, as long as you can complete the exercise comfortably. The point is to get yourself moving. Tomorrow, you can add another minute. And then another the next day. If you get to a point where the exercise feels uncomfortable, back down—but don't give up. Keep increasing your time. Soon you'll be up to 10 minutes. Then 15. As you start to move more, your body will learn how to handle the stress of exercise. You'll be able to push yourself a little harder. You'll actually look forward to the challenge. But you won't get to that point if you push yourself too far in the beginning.

Make a commitment with yourself that you'll do a little exercise each day for the next month. Behavioral experts agree that it takes 21 days to erase old habits and replace them with new ones. If you've been taking these incremental steps toward fitness, by the time Week 3 rolls around, you'll be used to your new routine. Eventually, you'll start to look forward to your evening walk. Exercise will become less of something you *have* to do and more of something you *want* to do.

Scheduling and Accountability

Scheduling and accountability are two big tools in helping you develop the exercise habit. This goes back to two of Dorfman's five W's: *when* are you going to exercise, and *who* will you be exercising with?

Schedule your exercise time just as you would an appointment. Write it into your calendar or PDA. Many people enjoy exercising in the morning; it gets their blood

GET PSYCHED

"When I don't feel like exercising, I tell myself I'll just drive over to the park to get coffee. Then I'll see someone else out there walking and that's it, I'm out there, too." –*Lillian, Boston, Massachusetts*

pumping and gives them a psychological boost knowing their exercise is done for the day. Other people enjoy working out at lunchtime. A half-hour walk with a co-worker can be a great way to squeeze in exercise with a busy schedule. Still others like to exercise in the evening. It allows them to burn off the stress of the day.

Being accountable to someone other than yourself can also help turn exercise into a habit. If you know your neighbor is depending on your companionship during an evening walk, you'll probably be less likely to skip your exercise. If you sign yourself up for a 5K run in the future, this can put some positive pressure on your exercise program. There are all sorts of tricks to making yourself feel accountable. For example, when I decided to train for a triathlon, I let one of my friends know my plans. She, too, is doing the same triathlon and is thrilled to have someone join her. If I feel like slacking off on my training, I think about how disappointed she'll be on race day if I'm not ready to run, bike, and swim with her. That keeps me motivated.

How Much Exercise? In 2005, when the federal government released its new dietary guidelines, it also made a recommendation that to sustain weight loss in adulthood, Americans need moderate to vigorous exercise 60 to 90 minutes on most days of the week. That news was discouraging to a lot of people. But that's the ideal. If you're sedentary, any amount of exercise you start doing during the week is better than none at all. If you manage to work up to 30 minutes of moderate exercise every day, the same government guidelines say that's enough to ward off chronic disease.

WEB TALK: Take a small step toward better health and fitness at:

➤ www.smallstep.gov

Right now, when you're starting out, don't focus on those 60 or 90 minutes, or even on getting 30 minutes of exercise every day. That's something you can work up to. If you can only squeeze in 15 minutes a day, you're better off than the person who doesn't do anything at all. Lisa Dorfman, R.D., a sports nutritionist and licensed psychotherapist, as well as a competitive runner and triathlete, agrees. "You want to do anything that makes you breathe." Focus on what you can do *today* to improve your fitness, and the rest will fall into place.

What You Can Do

Whether you have 10 pounds to lose or 100, exercise helps you meet your weight-loss goals a lot easier than through diet alone. Not only does exercise help you burn calories faster, it also makes you look better, feel better, and live better.

- ☐ Before starting any fitness program, get a thorough physical exam with your M.D. Discuss your fitness plans with her, and follow any recommendations she gives.
- ☐ Look for small ways to incorporate fitness into your life. Buy a pedometer and track how much you walk every day. Look for ways to increase the number of steps you take the following day.
- ☐ Enjoy walking but dislike cold weather? Many malls around the country host "mall walkers" early in the morning. You can walk comfortably in a climate-controlled environment—for free!
- ☐ Look into low-cost community education programs where you can take classes in everything from yoga and tai chi to water aerobics and modern dance.
- ☐ Consider working with a trained fitness professional to help you develop an exercise plan you'll stick with.

☐ If you feel self-conscious about exercising, remember: no one is as interested in your weight as you are. Keep in mind that other people are busy worrying how *they* look, so they probably aren't spending a lot of time watching you. Focus on how exercise makes you feel rather than how you might look to others.

Sticking With the Plan

Y ou've been dieting for 1, 2, or 3 months—or maybe for a year. You're beginning to notice some things— some positive things—about dieting. You're also noticing some negatives.

It's time to enjoy all the good things you've learned about losing weight and learn how to incorporate those things into your new life. It's also time to figure out how to head off the last-ditch saboteurs to your diet plan. If you're getting bored with your food choices, how can you spice things up—literally and figuratively?

Healthier Habits Come with Time

Changing your eating and exercise habits can feel unnatural at first, but over time, living with the changes gets easier. Remember when you first learned a new skill such as riding a bicycle? The first few times you sat on a bicycle seat felt unnatural. You probably fell down a lot. It was exhausting. You even probably wanted to give up a few times. But as your muscles got used to the activity and your balance improved, bicycling got easier. You didn't fall down as much. You could pedal and stay upright. Soon you began to enjoy the experience. Now you probably jump on a bike and don't even think about what you have to do to stay upright.

The same goes with developing healthy habits. At first, you struggled with meal planning and buying the correct foods for your diet. If you've never cooked your own meals before, all the food prep may have felt unnatural. You resented the time you had to spend prepping your meals and snacks because it took you away from other activities you enjoy. But within a few weeks or maybe even days, cutting up vegetables for a work snack became just another thing you did in the morning, like brushing your teeth. Plus, you started seeing the results of your efforts. You may be 10 or 20 pounds lighter, which reinforces your new habits.

Or perhaps you tried making healthier substitutes for food you enjoy. Take milk, for example. You may be used to drinking whole milk, and now you're trying to reduce your fat intake by

you're not alone

At 5'3", I weighed 179 pounds in December 2003. A few months earlier I had started working out at a gym with a personal trainer to strengthen my body and quit putting my back out—an old injury further irritated by three car accidents. I could feel muscle development but couldn't see it, so in January 2004, I started keeping a food diary to watch what I was eating and track overall caloric intake. With two strength-training sessions a week, plus four or five cardio sessions, I started to lose weight. By April, I started to run for the first time in 30 years. A little at first, but I worked up to 3- and 6-mile runs. By July, I was down to 161 pounds.

The trainers are great, as are the other clients in this small gym. But mostly, the results are the incentive. As for food, I don't eat as much, particularly things such as bread and pasta, but I am eating more protein. I used to eat at least a loaf of bread a week; now I put bread in the freezer and typically use a loaf a month. Breakfast is mostly

buying 1 percent fat or nonfat milk. It tastes watery at first, and nothing like the whole milk you love. But eventually you get used to the nonfat version—so used to it that now a mouthful of whole milk seems disgusting to you. Psychologist James O. Prochaska, Ph.D., of the University of Rhode Island, often asks dieters in his lecture audiences, "How many of you are confident you'll never go back to whole milk?" Most of the audience raises their hands. Eventually, giving up an old habit stops being a struggle for dieters.

A study conducted at the University of Newcastle on Tyne in the United Kingdom followed 200 schoolchildren over 20 years. The results of the study, published in the academic journal *Appetite* in 2004, were surprising and countered popular opinion. As adults, the subjects ate twice the amount of fruits and vegetables and less fats and sugars, suggesting that diets *do* get healthier over time. However, the same study showed

high-protein and -fiber Kashi cereal with soy milk, a piece of fruit, plus a soy latte. For lunch, I'll eat almost anything—typically eaten out, but not fast food. For dinner, sometimes it's a real meal, or sometimes it's just cottage cheese and fruit. Depends on what's in the fridge and how late I get home.

My routine today is two weight-training sessions (20 to 25 minutes each) and five or six cardio sessions. Some days I'll do 3- or 6-mile runs; other days I'll do the treadmill with a 10 percent incline (20 to 30 minutes), or I'll use an elliptical trainer, where I'll do 20 minutes with sprints interspersed. My weight has gotten as low as 152 but is

currently 157. I went from pushing the limits of a size 16, to thinking about buying size 10 jeans. I have muscle definition, haven't had colds or the flu in two years, sleep well, and don't have any aches and pains worth mentioning. My total cholesterol is down 40 points. —*Stephanie, 48, Seattle, Washington, lost 22 pounds*

that many adults had perceived barriers to good eating—they thought they didn't have time to prepare healthful meals or cut up vegetables, for example. However, the study showed it was a perceived lack of time rather than actual free time influencing their food choices. So there's hope for you yet.

Improved Eating Habits One of the benefits of sticking to a long-term weight-loss program is that you'll find your eating habits changing. Because you start repeating those habits over and over again, they become easier for you.

For example, when you were overweight and stressed, you may have reached for the nearest snack: a candy bar or a bag of salty, greasy potato chips. Then you started your diet. Reaching for your weight-loss journal probably felt strange at first when you were dealing with stress, but eventually it got easier. Now when you're stressed, you no longer reach for food. Instead, you go out for a walk or you chew on a carrot rather than crunchy chips.

You also might start sitting down for meals instead of eating on the run. Food may even taste better to you for many reasons: you linger over it longer so your stomach has time to tell your brain you're satisfied, or you may feel fuller on less food when you learn better portion control.

To keep up your new and improved eating habits, be sure you have all the tools you need to maintain them. If you're finding it difficult to keep your veggies chopped up and ready to go, look at your physical environment. Do you have sharp knives, an easy-to-use peeler, and a cutting board at the ready? Plenty of plastic storage containers or resealable bags? Enough room in the refrigerator? A few simple changes or additions to your tools and space can make a huge difference in your motivation.

New Tastes, New Horizons One of the things I've spent a lot of time talking about is how hard dieting is for most people. Yet developing new eating habits brings a multitude of gifts to dieters. They often discover new foods they enjoy or learn how to cook after a lifetime of eating convenience foods. Or they become more adventurous in their eating as they look to other cultures for foods.

Dieting forces you to get creative about food. If you enjoy cooking, you may find you enjoy the challenge of coming up with new recipes for your family or spouse. Try to make your diet an adventure. Losing weight can be a great way to learn about new foods:

- Revisit foods you disliked as a child because your tastes have probably changed over time. My mother used to force me to eat Brussels sprouts—a vegetable that's a nutritional powerhouse for dieters. As an adult, I tried them roasted in a bit of olive oil and sea salt and was surprised by their mellow, earthy—and delicious—taste! What is it for you? Broccoli? Mushrooms? Pinto beans?

- Experiment with foods from different cultures. Asian food, for example, offers many dishes made with leafy green vegetables and soy.

- Pick up new foods at the grocery store. If you enjoy seafood, purchase fish you've never eaten before, such as skate, halibut, or red snapper. Like ground beef? Choose ground buffalo, which is naturally leaner than ground beef but just as tasty.

- Look for food substitutions that give you some of the qualities your old favorites offered. People on low-carb diets, for example, have become masterful at turning

199

diet no-no's such as crème brûlée and pancakes into diet-friendly versions.

- Take a cooking class. Many communities offer classes that focus on preparing healthy meals or eating on a diet. You can learn some new recipes and cooking techniques that will make dieting easier for you.

- If you find a healthful food you enjoy, find different ways of preparing it so you don't get bored. Chicken breasts are a good example. They're a terrific food choice for people following a high-protein, low-fat diet, and you can prepare them in literally hundreds of ways so they don't get "stale."

- Experiment with herbs and spices. If you're watching your salt intake, for example, use herbs and spices judiciously to perk up most meals.

Sleep: Your Secret Weapon

America is a tired nation. We're getting less sleep than ever—some experts estimate Americans get less sleep than they did a century ago. Because we're also getting heavier as a nation, scientists are exploring a possible link between sleeplessness and obesity.

Does being overweight or obese cause disruptive sleep? Or does the cutting back on sleep cause some people to gain weight? What researchers do know is that when dieters lack sleep, they tend to reach for food more often than people without disordered sleep patterns.

In one study reported in the January 10, 2005, issue of the *Journal of the American Medical Association,* Robert D. Vorona, M.D., from the Eastern Virginia Medical School in Norfolk and his colleagues showed that obese and overweight patients reported sleeping less than their peers with normal body mass indexes

(BMIs). As total sleep time decreased, BMIs increased, except in the severely obese group. The authors wrote, "Our findings suggest that major extensions of sleep time may not be necessary, as an extra 20 minutes of sleep per night seems to be associated with a lower BMI."

In another study conducted at the Yale School of Medicine, researchers found a possible link between obesity and lack of sleep. In an article published in the April 2005 issue of the scientific journal *Cell Metabolism,* the authors Tamas Horvath, associate professor in the departments of obstetrics, gynecology and reproductive sciences (Ob/Gyn) and neurobiology, and Xiao-Bing Gao noted that certain neurons in the hypothalamus area of the brain are easily excited and stimulated by stress. They believe that these neurons, when stimulated, trigger sleeplessness, which triggers overeating. Horvath found both obesity and insomnia result from the same overactive brain system. Therefore, he wrote, "People with weight and sleep problems could benefit from cutting back on stressful aspects of their lives, rather than trying to specifically medicate either insomnia or obesity."

WEB TALK: Read more about sleep disorders at the National Center on Sleep Disorders Research's website at:

www.nhlbi.nih.gov/sleep

How can you improve your sleep during weight loss?

- Stick to a regular sleep schedule. Go to bed and wake up at roughly the same times, even on the weekends when you're tempted to stay up later or sleep in longer.
- If you like to eat at night, try to curtail the habit. Going to bed with a full stomach can cause you to sleep less soundly, or prevent you from falling asleep quickly.

- Avoid drinking alcohol or caffeine at night. Alcohol disrupts sleep cycles, and caffeine is a stimulant, which can keep you from falling asleep.

- If you simply cannot get a good night's sleep—you wake up regularly or have trouble falling asleep—consult your doctor and get a thorough medical exam. Sleeplessness or night waking can be signs of more serious conditions, such as sleep apnea or depression.

- If you exercise in the evening and have trouble falling asleep, try shifting your exercise to the morning. You may be stimulating your body too much before bedtime, making it hard for you to fall asleep.

Q & A

What is insomnia?

Approximately 60 million Americans experience insomnia each year. It tends to occur more often in older adults and affects 40 percent of women and 30 percent of men. According to the National Women's Health Information Center, a project of the U.S. Department of Health and Human Services, Office on Women's Health, people with insomnia experience one or more of the following symptoms:

- Difficulty falling asleep
- Waking up often during the night and having trouble going back to sleep
- Waking up too early in the morning
- Unrefreshing sleep

Insomnia is not defined by how many or few hours of sleep you get per night. Americans average 7 hours of sleep per night; but some people need more or get by just fine on less.

Eat Diet-Friendly Foods

When many people think "diet food," they think of an endless routine of celery, carrots, and cottage cheese. However, a great number of foods, many typically not thought of as diet foods, can be extremely beneficial for weight loss as well as improved health.

Although there's no one magic food that will melt away pounds, a great number of foods contain nutrients and chemical compounds found to help dieters lose or maintain weight. The composition of these foods can also affect common health conditions experienced by the overweight and obese, such as high blood pressure, heart disease, and certain cancers.

Calcium-Rich Foods The link between calcium intake and weight loss is exciting. Many studies in the past few years have shown that people who eat at least the minimum RDA of calcium experience greater weight loss than dieters who eat a diet low in calcium. Experts aren't yet sure if it's the intake of calcium or low-fat, calcium-rich dairy foods impacting weight loss. Weight loss might even occur because of the increase or combination of other chemicals with calcium.

Researchers at Purdue University found that higher calcium intakes may reduce overall levels of body fat and slow weight gain for women. They studied 54 women between the ages of 18 and 31 for 2 years and discovered that subjects who consumed calcium from dairy products such as milk, yogurt, and cheese rather than those who

GET PSYCHED

"Not only is it critical to keep your calcium levels high so you won't lose bone density, it will also help you maintain your muscle mass and increase your fat loss. A diet rich in low-fat dairy foods, like yogurt, can help make your weight-loss efforts easier." —*Michael Zemel, professor of nutrition, University of Tennessee*

got their calcium from nondairy sources or supplements seemed to reap the most weight-loss benefits. It is not yet clear whether the findings apply to women over 30. Says Dorothy Teegarden, assistant professor of foods and nutrition at Purdue, "This difference may be attributed to the fact that women who use nondairy sources would have to eat significant amounts of those foods to produce the effect, or it may suggest that there is something in milk that works to help regulate body weight."

If the findings are confirmed, researchers believe it may prompt new calcium-intake recommendations, especially from dairy resources. The recommended dietary allowance (RDA) of calcium for adults is 1,000 to 1,200 milligrams per day, depending on age. Most Americans, unfortunately, get nowhere near this amount of calcium in their diets. It's not too hard, however, even on a weight-loss diet, to improve your calcium consumption. You can meet these requirements by taking 1 (500-milligram) calcium supplement, drinking 1 cup of fat-free milk, eating 1 (8-ounce) serving of yogurt, and 1 (1-ounce) slice of cheese.

Keep in mind that excess protein, caffeine, and sodium in your diet can exacerbate calcium loss. If you're eating a high-protein diet, increase your consumption of calcium-rich foods, or if you consume a lot of caffeine, consider cutting your consumption. And of course, watch your salt intake, which also promotes water retention.

If you're on a high-protein diet, include calcium supplementation. Some research shows that a high-protein diet combined with supplementation increases bone mass density.

Eat calcium-rich foods with other foods that improve calcium absorption in the body. For example, vitamin C helps the body absorb more calcium; think about putting orange segments on your spinach salad, or drink calcium-fortified orange juice or vitamin C–fortified nonfat milk.

Likewise, calcium blocks the absorption of iron in the body, so avoid drinking milk with spinach, for example. Avoid taking your multivitamin with calcium supplements.

WEB TALK: Find the Food and Nutrition Center at the National Agricultural Library's recommendations on fluid intake at:

www.iom.edu/Object.File/Master/20/004/0.pdf

Water Water doesn't have any magical weight-loss powers, but good hydration has numerous benefits for dieters. First, water helps move waste products out of your body. When you're burning fat, you're creating a lot of toxins, so it's important to get them flushed out of your system. Water assists your cells with this important task.

When you're not drinking enough water, your body and brain can trigger your hunger mechanism. You may *think* you're hungry, but you're actually dehydrated. Drinking water throughout the day can prevent this false trigger from occurring and keep hunger at bay. Dehydration also causes headaches, muscle aches, dizziness, and nausea, all of which can be misinterpreted by the dieter as a need for food. Another signal you need to drink more water is when your urine is dark and concentrated.

One way to determine how much water to drink: divide your weight by two. The resulting number is the number of water in ounces you should drink each day. For example, if you weigh 140 pounds, you should aim to drink 70 ounces of water per day. If you're exercising or live in a hot climate, you may need to drink additional water to remain properly hydrated.

Other good points about water …

- The old wives' tale about ice water burning more calories is true: your body burns additional calories when it has to "warm up" ice water. You'll burn an additional 70 calories a day if you ingest ice water. Over time, those calories can add up to weight loss.

- If you're having trouble increasing the amount of water you drink each day, start slowly. Try drinking four glasses a day, then move to five, and so on. Or use the "3-2-1" rule to start out—three glasses in the morning, two in the afternoon, and one at night.

- Have trouble remembering to drink up? Create a screensaver on your computer that reminds you to take a water break. Or set a timer to go off every hour. Some people drink a glass of water after urinating.

Q&A

How much water should I drink each day?

Try to drink eight 8-ounce glasses of water, spreading consumption throughout the day to keep yourself consistently well-hydrated. There's some debate whether herbal teas, coffee, and diet soda can replace some of that water. Some nutritionists and M.D.s say that water should be in addition to your other beverages; others say you can substitute beverages for some of that water. The U.S. Department of Agriculture (USDA), which is responsible for determining RDAs of nutrients for Americans, includes all fluid sources in meeting its water-consumption recommendations.

Red Wine and Grapes First, the bad news: because red wine is an alcoholic beverage, it contains calories, so you must account for them in your diet. The human body converts alcohol into sugar—and sugar equals calories. If you're not using sugar for energy, your body converts it into fat. The alcohol in a glass of wine can stimulate your appetite and depress your nervous system. This means it can have the double whammy of increasing your appetite while depressing your body's ability to gauge hunger and may explain why some people get the "munchies" when they're drinking alcohol. And last, alcohol tends to stimulate the body's production of the hormone cortisol, and increased cortisol is linked to weight gain in the midsection.

Now for the promising news about red wine and weight loss. A short-term study conducted at Colorado State University showed that the consumption of red wine did not appear to contribute to weight gain. Researchers studied 14 healthy males over a 12-week period. Some subjects drank 2 glasses of red wine with dinner daily for 6 weeks and others abstained from drinking alcohol for 6 weeks. Halfway into the study and at the conclusion, the researchers measured body weight, percentage of body fat, skin-fold thickness, and resting metabolic rate, as well as glucose and insulin levels in the blood. No changes were noted in any of the participants whether they drank red wine or abstained from alcohol. The findings, which were written up in the March 31, 1997 issue of the *Journal of the American College of Nutrition*, also showed that moderate red wine consumption (less than 5 percent of an individual's daily calories) did not affect levels of glucose and insulin in the blood, which often increase with weight gain.

In another study using mice at Oregon State University, the Massachusetts Institute of Technology, and the University of Ottawa, researchers found that a gene called SIRT1 reduces the development of new fat cells and improves fat metabolism in existing cells. When cells were exposed to resveratrol, an anti-oxidant found in red wine as well as in some plants, there was a dramatic reduction in the conversion to fat cells and a lesser but still significant increase in the mobilization of existing fat.

Other studies have shown that drinking red wine in moderation—one or two 5-ounce glasses a day—may offer protective health benefits beyond weight loss. Nearly all dark red wines—

merlot, cabernet, zinfandel, shiraz, and pinot noir—contain resveratrol. Studies have shown that resveratrol has a positive effect on atherosclerosis (hardening of the arteries), heart disease, arthritis, and autoimmune disorders—all conditions suffered by a high number of patients suffering from overweight and obesity.

Scientists at the USDA have identified another compound in grapes that they believe shows promise in fighting cancer. The compound, pterostilbene, is similar to resveratrol. Dark-skinned grapes (such as red and blue-black) are likely to contain the most pterostilbene, while green grapes (also called white grapes) probably contain less. For reasons that are unclear, pterostilbene is not normally found in wine. Researchers suspect it may be because the substance is unstable in light and air, which makes it less likely to survive the wine-making process. So if you don't like wine, you can get health-protective benefits from eating dark-skinned grapes or grape juice. Resveratrol is also found in raspberries, mulberries, blueberries, cranberries, and peanuts.

The bottom line: red wine in moderation definitely has health benefits. If you really enjoy a glass of wine now and then, you may be able to incorporate it into a healthy weight-loss plan. However, it's important to note that everyone metabolizes alcohol differently. You may find that when you're trying to lose weight, even one glass of wine at night can have an effect on you. If you find your weight loss has stalled or it's getting more difficult for you to lose, you may have to take a fresh look at your alcohol consumption.

Water-Rich Foods Water-rich foods can help you "bulk up" your diet without bulking *you* up. These foods are also called low-energy-density foods. Per ounce, they have fewer calories than high-energy-density foods, but because they're high in water content, which gives them more bulk, they help you feel more full. For example, look at a 100-calorie serving of raisins, which is only $1/4$ cup, and compare it to a 100-calorie serving of grapes. Because the grapes have more water, you'll be able to eat $1^2/_3$ cups compared to the $1/4$ cup of raisins.

Research at Pennsylvania State University in 1999 showed that drinking water before and during meals doesn't reduce hunger or help you eat less to control your weight. The results of the study, which were published in the *American Journal of Clinical Nutrition* in October 1999, showed it was more important for dieters to consume water-rich foods to control appetite. Dieters then don't have to limit portion size as much because the body's satiety centers don't notice the lower calories; it's satisfied with the extra bulk.

Barbara Rolls, Ph.D., who worked on the 1999 Pennsylvania State University study, wrote a book called *The Volumetrics Weight-Control Plan: Feel Full on Fewer Calories*, which explains the concept of eating low-energy-density foods to lose weight. Following are some of her tips for incorporating these foods into your diet:

- Reduce the energy density of foods you love. You can make chili, for example, with leaner meats and bulk it up with tomatoes, mushrooms, and other vegetables without increasing calories.

- Snack on foods with high water and fiber content. Some people think pretzels are healthy, but they contain very little water and little to no fiber. You get more water and fiber—and thus bulk—with an apple.

- Eat a bowl of low-calorie soup before lunch and dinner to help fill you up.

Chocolate First, let's be honest: you cannot eat a regular diet of chocolate bars and expect to lose weight. However, moderate consumption of chocolate can be part of an effective weight-loss strategy for many people—especially if you feel you cannot live without chocolate for the rest of your life!

Chocolate is high in fat and calories, yes. Yet one third of the saturated fat found in chocolate is made of stearic acid, which does not raise LDL cholesterol (the "bad" cholesterol), unlike other saturated fats. This is because the liver converts stearic acid into oleic acid, a monounsaturated ("good") fat. Oleic acid also makes up another third of the total fat found in chocolate.

Scientists have found more than 300 naturally occurring chemicals in chocolate, some of which have been shown to have tremendous health benefits. Chocolate contains phenols, the same antioxidants found in red wine, and studies have shown these phenols prevent plaque buildup on the artery walls. The darker the chocolate, the more phenols it contains. Chocolate also has significant amounts of magnesium and phosphorus, which your body needs. Research shows it has far less caffeine than commonly believed, and much less than coffee.

GET PSYCHED

"People thank me all the time for telling them that chocolate is good for them. And really it is. I eat a little bit of chocolate every day." —*Joe Vinson, Ph.D., chocolate researcher at the University of Scranton, Pennsylvania, quoted in* Psychology Today, *January/February 2003*

If you simply cannot give up chocolate, you can incorporate it into a successful weight-loss plan. For example ...

Drink hot cocoa prepared with nonfat milk and a sweetener such as Splenda to cut back on calories. A recent study done at Cornell University shows that a cup of hot cocoa contains more antioxidants than a glass of red wine or a cup of tea. Moreover, you'll boost your calcium intake with the milk!

Give dark chocolate a co-starring role in desserts to reduce the amount of fat you ingest. For example, dip strawberries in dark chocolate, or swirl chocolate sauce into nonfat yogurt.

Choose dark, bittersweet chocolate over milk chocolate. The higher the cocoa content, the more antioxidants you'll get in your diet.

Developing a Reward System

Some people believe the reward of weight loss should be the actual weight loss. If they can remain motivated for months or possibly years by working for that ultimate reward, more power to them. But for most of us, a simple reward for good effort can help sustain momentum on a diet, whether you have 10 pounds to lose or 100.

Many commercial weight-loss programs recognize how effective rewards can be. At Weight Watchers meetings, for example, members who make their 10 percent weight-loss goals receive a keychain. When they make their goal weights, they get their goal weight charm, and dieters who maintain their weight over a period of time get another charm. If you join Weight Watchers online, you can earn a little star next to your member name for every 5 pounds you lose. That tiny star is enough to motivate many members to continue on their diets!

Rewards don't have to be expensive, nor do they have to be tied to the actual weight you've lost. If you find it difficult to drink your eight glasses of water every day, reward yourself with a new paperback mystery when you maintain your daily water intake for a week.

Set up some rewards for your weight-loss milestones. I know dieters who've treated themselves to a snazzy new outfit for every size they drop. (You have to buy clothes anyway; why not something you really like?) Other ideas include professional manicures and pedicures, a new CD or DVD, a visit to a local museum, or an addition to a personal collection. One thing to avoid: food rewards. The psychology between food and good behavior is probably twisted-up enough in your head without adding a new layer of confusion to it.

Write down your rewards so you can see them frequently. Some people even like to create collages of their rewards. For example, someone who has promised himself a trip to Europe might find a collage of magazine photos of Paris, London, and Rome very inspiring.

The flip side of rewards is punishments, and it's generally not a good idea to punish yourself when you haven't met a goal or when you've "goofed." A better strategy is to examine what went wrong and ask yourself how you'll improve next time. Not getting the reward you'd planned is punishment enough, and it'll be all the sweeter when you finally do earn it.

Looking at Alternative Therapies

When a local acupuncturist approached Elena Ramirez's weight-control clinic at the University of Vermont about offering her services to participants, Ramirez had to decline. Her program is data-driven, and according to Ramirez, the data just wasn't there to show that acupuncture was effective for weight loss.

That said, many dieters do turn to alternative therapies such as acupuncture, massage, and hypnosis to augment weight-loss programs. They find these nontraditional treatments help them in ways that may not be measurable by science. A weekly massage, for example, may reduce your stress and get you more in touch with your body. If a few sessions of hypnosis make you feel more determined to stick to your healthy eating habits, then go for it!

Some of these therapies are covered under insurance plans, but the majority are not. To get a clear picture about how much the treatment will cost you, ask the therapist how many sessions you'll need to attend to see improvement. A massage may make you feel like dancing the first time you get one; acupuncture may not have any effect on your appetite until weeks later. If your acupuncturist tells you most dieters show reduced appetite after 3 weeks of treatment and you're not seeing any change in your life, you'll have to re-evaluate the program's effectiveness and cost.

Many dieters find success with tapes and books of affirmations. Affirmations are phrases you repeat over and over to yourself. They are positive sayings and are phrased in the present tense. Some examples …

> *I am getting fitter and healthier every day.*
>
> *I feel great when I'm moving.*
>
> *I love my body, and I'm doing the best I can to take care of it today.*

Many psychologists and self-help experts believe that as you repeat positive statements to yourself, your brain begins to believe them and acts in ways that support the positive message, rather than against it. That is, if you tell yourself a hundred times a day you eat a healthful, low-fat diet, your behaviors will soon follow.

Affirmations can be especially helpful to people who are plagued by low self-esteem or who speak of themselves disparagingly. If you often put yourself down by telling yourself "I'm a fat slob with no control" or "I'll never lose this weight. Why bother?" you may want to give affirmations a try.

Some people feel strange repeating positive, uplifting affirmations to themselves, especially if they've spent most of their lives speaking badly of themselves. Just try it! If you notice you're telling yourself things such as, "I'll never lose this weight," change the voice to say, "I am losing weight." If you feel funny saying these phrases out loud, you can think them instead or write them down in your journal. Make a tape of yourself saying these affirmations, and listen to them while you're walking or doing housework. Most bookstores and libraries have large selections of affirmational tapes, some written specifically for people trying to lose weight.

GET PSYCHED

"Losing weight and getting healthy is a step-by-step process. It can be an adventure that leads you to alternatives you haven't considered before."
—*Susan Jeffers, Ph.D., author of* Feel the Fear and Do It Anyway

Overcoming Setbacks

We all suffer setbacks—it's part of the human condition—so it's unrealistic to expect as a dieter you'll be "perfect" and not experience them. Setbacks are usually temporary, and they can provide you with a valuable learning tool.

When you find yourself in the midst of a dietary setback—you've gained weight during school exams or you find yourself eating more sweets than usual—grab your weight-loss journal and answer these questions:

- What situation or event led to this setback?
- How did I respond to the setback? (Be gentle on yourself. This isn't the time to beat yourself up—simply be objective about your responses.)
- How can I handle a similar setback the next time it happens?

Write down your answers in your weight-loss journal so you'll have something to review next time a setback threatens to knock you off-course.

If you've come this far, don't let a temporary derailment turn into a permanent one. Look at your progress to date. Pat yourself on the back for the effort you've made up to now. And then get back on your eating plan.

Work Your Vices for Success

We're humans. We're imperfect. No matter how hard we try, we'll always have personality traits that work against our better intentions. I talked about how to work on psychological barriers to weight loss in earlier chapters, but this is where I'm going to talk about using vices you simply can't change to further your weight-loss goals. It's the "if you can't beat them, join them" section of the book!

Why do today what you can put off until tomorrow? Many dieters are very good at procrastinating. "I'll start my diet and exercise program tomorrow." "I'll start a food diet next week." "As soon as I get through this stressful time at work, I'll think about losing weight."

If you're a skillful procrastinator, try using procrastination in creative ways. For example, if you're really craving chocolate and your head tells you to really indulge, tell yourself, "I'm not going to eat any chocolate for an hour." During that hour, drink some water and have some other kind of snack. If, when the hour is up, you still want that chocolate, go ahead and have a small piece.

GET PSYCHED

"I let myself watch *General Hospital*, but only at the gym. It gave me the incentive to go work out *and* it made me work out longer. Typically I'd go on the treadmill or bike for a half-hour, but I wanted to see the whole show, so I'd keep on going for a full hour." *–Patti, Stratford, Connecticut*

Take a little bit of action now on something you're putting off. For example, if you're putting off joining a gym, spend 10 minutes compiling a list of local gyms in the area. Tomorrow, spend another 10 minutes calling them. If you feel like spending more than 10 minutes on the project, go for it!

After a long day at the office or when the kids go to bed, many adults like nothing better than to plop down on the couch and watch television. Many studies have linked children and television viewing—even as little as 2 hours a day—to overweight and obesity, so this may be a vice you've picked up from your own childhood.

If you watch a lot of television, or engage in a lot of other sedentary activities during the day, try ...

- Making it a rule not to eat in front of the television. If you want to eat, turn the TV off, get yourself a snack, and eat it at the kitchen table.

- Stretching exercises every hour, especially if you sit down a lot on the job. Regular stretching promotes alertness, gets your blood flowing, and possibly prevents a dangerous condition called deep vein thrombosis (DVT), which is when a blood clot develops in a deep vein in the leg, breaks loose, and lodges in the lungs.

- Doing butt squeezes when you're commuting.

- Limiting television viewing time. Watch only those television shows you enjoy, and do something to keep your mind off snacking: do sit-ups, pedal on your exercise bicycle, or walk on a treadmill.

What You Can Do

You can do a lot to remain positive and upbeat and squeeze every bit of enthusiasm into your diet:

☐ Remind yourself that dieting and healthful eating are new skills, and like all skills, they take time to master. They also *do* get easier with time.

☐ Bring a sense of adventure to your weight-loss program. What new foods can you try? How can you make your food taste better without adding more fat or calories?

☐ Remember—dieting isn't easy for anyone. Take it slowly, go gentle on yourself, and adopt a philosophy of continuing improvement.

☐ Think about the fun ways you can reward yourself for the goals you've achieved. Get creative. What is something you'd really enjoy and look forward to when you reach some of your milestone goals?

☐ If you enjoy "no-no" foods such as wine and chocolate, figure out a way to incorporate them into your weight-loss plan without jeopardizing your goals.

☐ Consider augmenting your weight loss with alternative therapies that make you feel good. Massage, acupuncture, hypnosis, and biofeedback help some dieters in mysterious ways.

Tips from the Successful

As the saying goes, "If you want to know how to do something, watch someone who knows how to do it." Noticing how other people interact with food and approach health and exercise can be a great learning tool as you're working on your own weight loss. According to researchers, naturally slim people have a number of common habits—and formerly overweight people have adopted those habits, with success. Not every "trick of the trade" is healthy or even safe, so use good judgment when you're observing others.

Lessons from the "Naturally Slim"

People who are "naturally slim" often don't get a fair shake. As with overweight and obese people, the naturally slim are regularly subject to assumptions about their size and rude comments about their weight. Up until my late 20s, I was one of the naturally slim. Friends, family members, and strangers would ask or comment:

> *How can you eat that and stay so skinny?*
>
> *Do you starve yourself to keep thin?*
>
> *You must have a fast metabolism.*

Don't worry, you'll be fat like me someday.

And the worst: *I hate you because you're thin.*

you're not alone

I grew up in central Vermont in the 1940s. When I was a kid, there were no organized sports outside of school—no soccer, no T-ball. The only thing vaguely exercise-related was roller skating on Friday nights. But we also didn't have television like they do today, or video games. We always spent a lot of time outdoors, hiking around the woods or swimming at a local swimming hole.

Neither of my parents had weight problems, which probably helps me a bit. My mother was a champion basketball player in high school. I don't remember her ever exercising, but she was always active. She didn't drive, so she walked everywhere—to the store for groceries, to the hospital for her nursing job. My father didn't exercise either, but he was always out in the woods, hunting with his dogs. I don't remember either of them ever sitting around doing nothing.

I've always been active like my parents. I played basketball in high school, and I played on local teams as an adult. Then I took up running in my 30s, and eventually became a marathoner. I still run, but I no longer compete in marathons. Now I'm into cycling, which keeps me in shape in the spring, summer, and fall. During the winter, I don't really do too much, which is why my weight goes up to around 190. When spring comes and I start cycling again, it drops down to 179.

If I like a food, I eat it. If I don't like it that much, I don't eat it. That's my eating philosophy. I don't eat much during the day, especially in the mornings. But sometimes I'll go out to breakfast with my wife and get eggs Benedict because I like eggs Benedict a lot. And sometimes I'll finish her plate, too. When I'm full, I don't eat any more, no matter how good it tastes. That's it. I'm done.

I don't know what being overweight feels like, and I'm sure it's not easy to lose weight in general. But it's also not that complicated. People seem to make it more complicated than it really is. You have to burn more calories than you take in—you move more and you eat less. That's my secret. *—John, 65, Bethel, Vermont*

It's important to get past the envy or anger of someone who is naturally slim. You can't assume they don't work as hard as you to maintain their weight. Sure, some people can eat whatever they want, sit around all day, and never gain an ounce—most of them are called teenagers! But far more "healthy weight" people engage in habits and behaviors that promote and help them maintain their healthy weight. All you need to do is open your eyes to them.

For example, Toni M., a 38-year-old mother from Chicago, had a recent eye-opening experience when she served as a bridesmaid in a wedding. She had eaten all the food on her plate at the reception and then looked over at the slim bridesmaid sitting next to her, who was only about a third of the way through her meal. "And it just struck me she ate at a much slower pace than I did," said Toni. The take-away lesson? Slim people tend to eat more slowly, savoring their food and giving their stomachs time to signal their brains when they're satisfied.

People who are "naturally thin" tend to share these qualities:

- They take small, slow bites and chew their food well before swallowing.
- They eat when they're hungry, and they stop eating when they're satisfied.
- They take the focus off the food in front of them, often engaging in conversation or even putting down their utensils to take a break from eating.
- If they're focused on the food in front of them, it's all they focus on. They're not looking at someone else's plate, silently thinking, *I hope she eats slowly so I can get that last piece of pizza.* They tend not to care or even notice how much other people are eating.

- They eat whatever they want, whenever they want it. But with this in mind, they usually self-regulate the amount they eat, eating only until they're satisfied. If they do "pig out," they usually make up for it the next day by eating less or working out harder.

- They do not label food as "bad" or "good." Rather, they see food as "something I enjoy eating" or "something I don't enjoy eating." Within those parameters, they make decisions about how much to eat and when to eat it.

- They understand their healthy weight isn't a free ride. They usually work to maintain it, although many people aren't around to see the hard work— they just see the results.

GET PSYCHED

"When traveling, I try to convert my love of food into a form of exercise. Before choosing where to have lunch or dinner, I first check out every restaurant within about a half-mile radius—looking at their menus posted in the windows and getting a general feel for the place. As a result, I may wind up doing a mile or more of walking before eating, but it doesn't feel like exercise, because I'm having the fun of comparing restaurants, making sure I don't overlook any, whether for myself or for both me and my wife."
—Peter, New York, New York

Next time you're around someone who is a healthy, normal weight, watch them closely. What is their relationship with food? Do they eat it slowly? Do they look like they're enjoying their meals? If you're eating with them, follow their eating pace, especially if they're a "slow eater." Do you notice any difference in how you feel after the meal?

Compile your observations in your weight-loss journal. Don't get discouraged if you meet a mother of three who insists she eats like a horse all day and that her six-pack abs are "heredity." There *are* some people in this world who don't want you to see their sweat. Move on to someone who doesn't mind getting real with you.

you're not alone

Around 10 years ago, give or take a few years, my father was diagnosed with coronary artery disease. He had to radically change his diet or else think about surgery. He ended up going on an extremely low-fat diet.

I decided to make easy changes now so I didn't have to make drastic changes later. I was in my early 30s and not overweight, but heart disease runs in my family. I didn't cut calories—I just wanted to change the mix of what I was eating, so I cut out high-fat foods.

Being from the Midwest, I grew up eating butter, red meat, bacon—a lot of fat. I remember eating warm bread with melted butter practically dripping off it. I loved the stuff. But I gave it up, even baked goods loaded with butter. What you don't realize is that your tastes may change—mine certainly did. Now I could never eat butter.

Not only did I give up butter, but I stopped eating the skin off chicken, something else I enjoyed. No more bacon or sausage, and I also cut back on sweets. I would never drink soda, for example. I ask myself, *Would I ever pour myself a glass of water, dump sugar in it, and drink it?* I eat very few sweets. Honestly, I'd like to and could probably eat 10 times more than I do, but I would gain weight, so I don't.

It's easy to think thin people are thin by nature, not by their actions, but it's certainly not true in my case. I suspect those "lucky folks" are few and far between. *—Scott, 41, Michigan*

When I was struggling with overweight after the birth of my son, I met a woman at my local gym who was two years older than I was and who had recently given birth. Moreover, this was her second child. She looked amazing! Her skin was glowing, her arms and legs were toned, and much to my dismay, her stomach was firm. She wasn't skinny, but she sure looked fit and firm, especially after having two kids!

After I got over my envy, I approached her and complimented her on her appearance. She seemed to appreciate my compliment, and she shared with me how she'd lost her "baby weight" and regained her shape. She happened to be a fitness trainer, which had helped her stay in shape during pregnancy and tone up afterward, but she also ate a diet rich in fruits and vegetables, drank lots of pure water, and avoided empty carbs. Her advice was "everything in moderation, but lots of the healthy stuff."

Lessons from Successful "Losers"

You can certainly learn many skills and tips from people who have never been overweight. But more important for you are the people who have been overweight or obese, often for most of their lives, but who've managed to lose their weight and remain at a healthy weight.

You can't assume everyone who's at a healthy weight has always been at a healthy weight. I was teaching a class during the spring of 2005. One of my students was a slender, 50-something blonde who looked as though she'd never had a weight problem in her life. I mentioned during my class that I was writing a book on the psychology of successful weight loss. During a break, she showed me a picture of herself, taken maybe 10 or 15 years before. The woman in the picture looked to be more than 200 pounds. She didn't at all resemble the petite woman standing next to me. I was astounded.

When you meet someone who has lost weight and kept it off, learn from them. What did they do to lose weight? What was difficult for them? How did they remain motivated? Do they still have to struggle with food, exercise, and temptation? How

GET PSYCHED

"Reading the stories of other big losers keeps me inspired. One of my favorites is *Thin for Life* by Anne Fletcher, in which Fletcher tells the stories of men and women who've lost major amounts of weight and kept it off. Whenever I need a little extra motivation or some good new tips, I flip it open and read a chapter. Works every time!" –*Melody, Ames, Iowa*

has being at a healthy weight impacted or changed their life or their health? Often their stories can be inspiring, especially if you're at a rough point in your own weight loss, such as when you're battling diet fatigue or working through a plateau.

Diet and Weight Data collected by the NWCR have shown that long-term weight maintainers share certain dietary characteristics:

The average subject in the database has lost about 60 pounds and has kept it off for 5 years, blowing the myth that it's impossible to beat "yo-yo" dieting. In fact, the majority of maintainers report they had been on dozens of diets before losing their weight permanently.

Eighty-nine percent of the people in the registry reported they used a combination of dietary and exercise changes to lose their weight; not one or the other. And 88 percent of registrants report they continue to watch what they eat and exercise regularly.

Eighty-eight percent of the registrants report they limit certain types of food; 44 percent reduce portion sizes; and 44 percent count calories.

Half the weight maintainers lost their weight through a formal program such as Weight Watchers, Jenny Craig, or a university weight-management program. The other half lost their weight on their own.

Two thirds of the people in the database were overweight or obese as children, and 60 percent report a family history of overweight or obesity.

Registrants report that they continue to consume a less energy-dense, low-fat diet even though they're no longer "dieting." Women report eating an average of 1,306 calories per day, while men consume an average of 1,685 calories per day. They report 56 percent of daily calories come from carbohydrates, 19 percent come from protein, and 25 percent come from fats. Few maintainers report losing or maintaining weight on a low-carbohydrate diet.

Subjects who lost weight through a program such as Weight Watchers versus subjects who lost weight on their own reported following diets that were similar to the commercial programs—that is, the diets were low in fat and their intake of selected nutrients such as iron, calcium, and vitamins A, C, and E were similar.

The most common food behaviors adopted by weight maintainers were watching the percentage of fat calories they consumed each day, eating a variety of foods, and controlling portion sizes.

When metabolic rates are measured, maintainers have similar resting metabolic rates to "normal weight" people not in the database, suggesting that metabolic rates can and do change.

An overwhelming number of long-term weight maintainers eat breakfast. Seventy-eight percent report eating breakfast every day, while only 4 percent report never eating breakfast. And breakfast-eaters report slightly more physical activity than non-breakfast-eaters.

GET PSYCHED

"I walked 6 or 7 days a week for a very long time. It became an ingrained habit, which helped to shed the pounds. I still walk about 4 or 5 miles a day 5 days a week."
—Jennifer N., Jacksonville, Florida, maintaining a 40-pound weight loss for 2 years

Exercise The majority of NWCR subjects exercised to help lose weight, and continue exercising to maintain weight loss. The database also shows …

Walking is the preferred exercise of most respondents, with aerobic dancing coming in second. This shows that a basic form of exercise can be just as effective at maintaining weight as more complicated or demanding exercise programs.

Seventy-two percent of registrants meet or exceed the American College of Sports Medicine's minimum exercise guideline to participate in 30 minutes of moderate-intensity exercise on most days. They burn, on average, up to 2,700 calories a week through exercise, which translates into an hour a day.

Behavior Registrants at the NWCR have adopted many behaviors that have helped them maintain their weight loss:

They are excellent at self-monitoring their weight. Contrary to a lot of expert advice, weight maintainers weigh themselves often. They also continue to record what they eat each day, and many keep a journal. This kind of self-monitoring suggests that they are able to correct "slips" early, before they escalate into weight regain.

These weight maintainers say that losing weight was hard work, but they've found the rewards have been worth it. They also report that keeping the weight off gets easier with time.

Maintainers continue to receive support, even though they're no longer actively "losing." They may check in with a support group or keep in touch with a health-care professional.

The majority of registrants participated in a variety of weight-management programs and diets before permanently losing their weight. When they were asked about their successful attempt, they said they had better reasons for losing weight this time around, such as social or health reasons. They also felt they were more committed with this attempt.

Weight maintainers report successful weight maintenance has improved their social interactions, health and well-being, and confidence.

What You Can Do

Look. Listen. Observe. Sometimes just keeping your eyes and ears open (while keeping your mouth firmly closed) can teach you a lot about getting and staying fit and trim. When you meet someone who has achieved weight loss goals similar to yours, take note. And put your own prejudices aside: you can also learn a lot from people who have never had weight issues.

☐ Make a point to observe and talk to people who are "naturally slim." How do they behave around food? What are their exercise habits like?

☐ If you make an observation about a "naturally thin" person, see if you can apply it to other people you've observed. If it seems like a reasonable conclusion, such as "naturally thin people tend to eat smaller portions than people I know who are overweight," this can be an *"Aha!"* moment you can learn from.

☐ Resist the urge to tease or joke with someone about how skinny they are, how much or little they eat, or how lucky they are to be so thin.

☐ Talk to people who've lost weight and kept it off for a long time. What do they say is the most important skill they've developed?

Dieting 911

You've been doing great on your diet. You're losing weight, your clothes are getting looser, and you may even be feeling better than you've felt in a long time. Way to go!

But everybody has them—situations that threaten to derail even the most diligent weight-loss plan. These situations can besmirch all the hard work you've accomplished to date—or, they can teach you something about yourself and make you an even stronger person, and more successful at weight loss.

If you've got a 911 dieting emergency, put down that dough-nut and relax—other dieters have gotten through similar emergencies, and so can you.

Emotional Eating

One of the toughest aspects of dieting is learning to divorce emotions from eating habits. It's fair to say most human beings have emotional attachments to food. These attachments can be as innocent as a happy childhood memory whenever you see a puff of pink cotton candy. They can be more complex, especially if you were rewarded or punished with food when you were "good" or "bad."

Many of us struggling with weight problems learned to equate food with comfort in our parents' arms. When we cried out as babies, we were consoled with a feeding. Later, as children, we were often rewarded with treats such as cookies, ice cream, or candy if we finished our meals or were "good" for our caregivers. If we were "bad," those treats were denied us.

As our parents' influence and ability to provide comfort diminished, we had to learn to comfort ourselves. You may have turned to food for that comfort—after all, it's what your parents used as a tool. If kids were picking on you at recess, ice cream after school made you feel better. If a girl turned down your invitation to the prom, an afternoon of stuffing yourself with your favorite hot dogs and French fries felt like it filled the emptiness in your soul.

GET PSYCHED

"One reason why people find it hard to lose weight is they have to give up food as comfort. So look at finding alternatives to the food as an adventure, an opportunity to discover other ways to comfort yourself."
—*Susan Jeffers, Ph.D., author of* Feel the Fear and Do It Anyway

The need to eat when we're feeling intense emotions isn't just psychological. Actually, complex chemical reactions occur when we ingest certain foods during emotional states. Chocolate is a good example. Chocolate contains a chemical in trace quantities called phenylethylamine, which humans produce naturally. This chemical is responsible for releasing dopamine in the pleasure center of our brain. When some people eat chocolate, they get the same pleasurable feelings they have after having an orgasm because the same chemicals are released.

you're not alone

I keep the picture in my purse because I want to remember what it feels like to weigh more than 260 pounds. I don't ever want to forget where I came from.

I came into the world weighing 11 pounds, 12 ounces. My family was Irish, so our meals in the 1950s were filled with potatoes and bread. I always looked at myself as being fat because I had those typical Irish features: a round face and a pug nose. But when I look back at pictures, I can see I wasn't fat. The fat was all between my ears.

In 1963, I joined the military so I could see the world. The following year, I was raped. My alcohol consumption went up, and I started getting promiscuous. Then I got pregnant and ended up married. Motherhood meant the world to me. I had eight children. With each pregnancy, I put on more weight. I also ate food to cope.

After 22 years, the marriage fell apart. I had four kids still left at home. My father and brother died of cancer within weeks of each other. I didn't have money to pay bills, but I had money for food. If I didn't, I put the food on a credit card. Eventually, I filed for bankruptcy. And I kept eating.

The day was December 14, 2002. In my freezer I had four Frisbee-sized oatmeal-raisin cookies I was saving for my grandchildren. I got up in the middle of the night and ate one, frozen. A half-hour later, I came out and ate another. A half-hour later, another. And by 6 A.M. I'd eaten all four cookies. I remember getting on my knees and crying.

I didn't go on a formal diet to lose more than 100 pounds. I cut out flour, sugar, and alcohol, and the weight started coming off. I joined a support group. I used little tricks with myself, like putting off eating a hot fudge sundae till the next day. When I woke up the next morning, I'd feel proud of myself. It boosted my self-esteem knowing I could stay away from the ice cream.

I've kept the weight off for 2 years, and I'm doing things today I'd never have done before. When I was heavy, I isolated myself: I didn't have nice clothes to wear, and I was afraid of what people thought of me. When I lost weight, I went back to school to learn medical terminology, and now I have a great job at a hospital. I volunteer as an usher at a local theater, and I travel. I date, and last year I walked a 5K race to support a local battered women's shelter. It felt wonderful.

I used to eat because of my problems. Today, if I thought a bag of chips or a gallon of ice cream would solve them, I'd run to the grocery store in a second. Now I know that kind of eating will only give me one more problem. *–Lillian, 60, Boston, Massachusetts*

Edward Abramson, Ph.D., a professor of psychology at California State University, Chico, studies the effects of emotions on eating behaviors and has published research on the effects of anxiety and boredom on eating. He agrees that emotional eating is something many dieters turn to for nurturing or soothing when they confront unpleasant emotions such as anger, depression, and loneliness. Unfortunately, part of being human means you will always have unpleasant emotions. The only things you can change are your reactions to those emotions and your reliance on food as comfort.

Abramson suggests a three-step plan for working with emotional eating:

1. First, identify what kind of emotional eater you are. Some people eat when they feel anxious or stressed. Others hit the cookie jar when they're bored or depressed. This is where a food journal can be helpful. When you write down how you're feeling whenever you get an urge to eat, you'll be able to discern your emotional patterns attached to food.

2. Get specific about how you're feeling as you reach for food. Note the times you're most vulnerable to emotional eating. Do you automatically reach for sweets at 3 p.m. when everything quiets down in your office? Are you sated or starving? What is going on around you? Note every detail in your journal.

3. After you start discerning patterns of your emotional eating behaviors, look for other ways to nurture yourself. For example, if you find yourself snacking every night in front of the television, look for other activities you can do instead. If you're watching television because you're bored, you could read or take up a new hobby. Or if you feel bored, rather than reach for food, you could call a friend or go for a run.

Emotional eating offers short-term relief for a long-term problem. A pint of maple walnut ice cream may make you feel good right now, but an hour from now, you'll be feeling remorseful about your eating. Compounding the situation is that you're probably reaching for foods that are not diet-friendly, because let's face it, how often do you reach for a salad or fruit when you're feeling down? Learn how to control your reactions to emotions without food, and you may, for the first time in your life, find weight loss much easier to attain.

Hunger Pangs

Hunger pangs provide a valuable service. They're a physical—often aural—indicator we need to eat. When we were babies, our hunger pangs triggered our cries so our parents could feed us. When the pangs stopped, we stopped eating. We were satisfied with the amount of food in our stomachs.

But somewhere along the way, many of us lose the ability to use our hunger pangs as a tool. For example, sometimes well-meaning caregivers, when they noticed we were upset, would give us food to calm us down. Or if we engaged in "good" behavior, we'd be rewarded with a cookie or another kind of treat. Eventually, the power of our hunger pangs was diminished by the emotional attachments we developed to certain kinds of food.

You may not have felt hunger pangs in years because you have learned to eat for other reasons besides hunger. Perhaps you eat whenever you feel stressed ... the act of putting food in your mouth calms you down, even if your stomach isn't empty. Or maybe you eat because you have a craving for a certain type of food—bread, cookies, or candy. You may eat when you feel weak or shaky, a sign of low blood sugar, so to get a quick boost of energy, you opt for something sugary and sweet. A few hours later, you're weak again—more sugar. Your body's hunger signals are so out of whack you're not even sure what hunger feels like anymore.

For some people, hunger is the sensation of growling and emptiness in their bellies—there may even be a growling, gurgling sound other people can hear across the room! Another person may feel it as a mild pain around the belly button. People who are extremely anxious may often confuse an anxious stomach with hunger, so it helps to look at your emotional state when determining how hungry you are. True hunger pangs can often feel uncomfortable, but despite the discomfort, they're an unmistakable signal that your body needs food.

GET PSYCHED

"I think of a hunger pang as a little fire in my stomach that burns calories. As long as I'm eating enough calories to stay healthy, this is a great way for me to deal with the occasional but inevitable pang." –Karin, Tennessee

Here's the tricky part: how much food? The problem a lot of dieters have is that they've been eating far more food than their bodies need to feel satisfied. They eat till they're stuffed and can barely move away from the table. Make a fist with your hand. That's as much as your stomach needs to feel satisfied, and maybe even less. It doesn't look like a lot of food, but it's plenty.

If you're out of touch with your body's signals to eat, it's time to get reacquainted with them. A useful tool is to use a "hunger scale" during the day to control your food intake. For example, if your stomach is empty and growling, you're at 0. If your stomach feels comfortable—not empty and not full—you're at 5. If you feel as though you've had a bit too much food, you can assign that feeling 7 or 8. And if you feel like you're about to burst, that's a 10.

Your goal is to eat only when you feel like you're at a 0 on the scale and eat till you're up to a 5. That's right, 5. You want to eat enough food to feel neither hungry nor stuffed.

Here's how to eat according to your body's signals ...

- Eat slowly, purposely, and consciously. Chew your food thoroughly and let all your senses enjoy the meal: the smell of the food, the texture and taste of it on your tongue, the feeling of it filling your stomach.

- Monitor how your body feels during the meal. How does your stomach feel after a few bites of food? Has the growling stopped? Is the drive to get food in your body diminishing as you eat?

- Eat with a friend or family member. When you eat alone, you tend to eat more food because you can focus all your attention on it. If someone's eating with you, chances are good you'll be talking and eating more slowly, thus giving your body a chance to fill up at a more reasonable pace.

- Allow yourself to eat whenever you feel hunger pangs. Don't try to ignore them; again, your body's telling you that you need food. However, choose a food that supports your weight loss—don't reach for something sugary or fatty. If you feel these pangs before a scheduled meal, an apple or a slice of cheese and a whole-grain cracker may be enough to satisfy your body.

> **GET PSYCHED**
>
> "I ask my children, 'Did you eat enough to be healthy?' I don't ask them if they're full, because fullness isn't the goal of the meal."
> —*Meredith, New Jersey*

- Practice taking and/or ordering smaller portions of food during meals. You usually can go back for more if you're still hungry.

- When you no longer feel hungry, simply stop eating. If you're at a restaurant, ask for a doggie bag and bring the rest of your meal home. If you're at home, put the leftovers in the fridge and skip dessert.

With time and patience, you'll soon be able to understand and work with your body's signals.

Cravings

There's a difference between an appetite and a craving. An appetite gives us desire for food. We all have certain appetites for certain foods, and that's perfectly natural.

A craving is a little different. A craving is an appetite gone wild. It's almost irrational, and certainly a lot of it is psychological. You may not even feel physically hungry, but still you crave the substance—chocolate, crunchy potato chips, or creamy peanut butter. Your brain won't shut up. The food you crave becomes your mind's mantra.

Some researchers believe we crave foods that contain nutrients or substances our body needs. For example, you may develop an intense craving for pasta or bread at some point because you have low blood sugar. Your body knows that a high-carb meal will give your body a quick boost. However, evidence also shows fluctuating levels of brain chemicals can trigger cravings. Serotonin, a neurotransmitter, is regulated by carbohydrate intake. When you take in too few carbs, serotonin levels are reduced, which triggers a physical desire for carbohydrate-rich food. In another example, coffee or soda consumption often creates strong cravings. In fact, someone who drinks a lot of caffeine-rich drinks often develops headaches because they haven't had their "morning hit."

Cravings can also develop through cultural associations. We associate some foods with our backgrounds and families, and eating them brings us comfort because they remind us of happy times. That's why they're called "comfort foods." My friend from Delhi craves her mother's rice pudding when she's back in India. Another friend craves her mother's sauerkraut whenever she's feeling homesick. Other people I know crave the macaroni and cheese or breakfast cereals of their childhoods, especially when they're stressed.

Still other people develop cravings for foods that are verboten. If you're on a formal diet that comes with a long list of foods you're not supposed to eat, you may develop cravings simply because it's human nature to want what you can't have.

If you struggle with cravings, it may be best for you to adopt a diet based on moderation. If you attempt to cut out carb-rich foods such as bread, for example, and for physical or psychological reasons you want a slice of bread now and then, you're going to be fighting an uphill battle by avoiding bread completely. Research suggests that stuffing yourself with another food to replace the food you actually crave rarely works. It's better to learn how to eat the food you crave *in moderation*. That way, your body and mind get a chance to relax. If you deny the craving completely, you run the risk of giving in and going overboard with it.

Dieting With a Family

You're on a diet, but your family's not. You may be eating more salads or less pasta, but nothing's changed for them. They still want their favorite meals and have no interest in changing their eating habits. How can you cope when you can't escape temptation in your own home?

If you're the person buying groceries in the house, you have it a little easier. Sometimes you can get away with making substitutions. It can be as simple as switching to lower-fat milk for your family or buying meats with lower fat contents—a ground chuck that's 90 percent lean versus 80 percent.

You can also talk to your family and explain how their food choices impact your diet. If you absolutely cannot have cookies around, ask family members to buy their own cookies and store them away from you. And keep in mind, if you're the person who's preparing meals, there's no law that says other family members have to eat foods different from yours, especially if you're practicing portion control. You can modify many favorite recipes for diets—and many times, your family will be no more the wiser. For example, if you're trying to cut fat and eat more veggies but your family insists on having Mom's lasagna on Friday nights, look for ways to trim fat. You can substitute low-fat ricotta and mozzarella cheeses for higher-fat versions and mix a box of chopped spinach into the cheese mixture.

Look at your diet as an opportunity to introduce and incorporate healthful foods into your family's diet. There's really no reason anyone in your family, even if they're in perfect shape, should be eating excess fat and sugars. Look for healthier substitutes for the foods your family likes. For example, rather than purchase high-fat corn chips for family snacks, you could try baked corn chips or bake whole-wheat pita breads till they're crispy. Keep in mind that some members of your family—namely young children in good physical condition—need dietary fat, so you may have to buy whole milk for them, as well as lowfat milk for yourself.

One thing you don't want to happen is to be caught short on your diet. If you're fighting a craving and your way of coping is to munch on celery with low-fat dip, you don't want to find out your daughter used the celery for her tuna salad sandwich and your husband ate the dip with his chips last night. Create a space for your healthy foods that's all yours. And be sure anything that's in a public area is clearly marked for your diet!

If you have children, you'll be giving them a lifelong gift by serving them the same healthful snacks you're eating on your diet—for example, a sliced apple with a small serving of cheese, yogurt, or some unsalted whole-grain pretzels. Ideally, over-processed, sugary, trans fat–laden snack foods should have no place in your family's diet.

Holidays and Special Events

Pick up a women's or health magazine around the winter holidays, and you'll find dozens of articles aimed at dieters. It's a rough season for those trying to lose weight, with the endless office parties, the rich holiday dishes we love the most, and plenty of alcohol to wash it all down.

And it's not just the food. We also have strong emotional attachments to holidays and special events. These special days can be stressful and bring out family conflicts. For many of us, holidays aren't the happy scenes played out in television commercials. So what do we do when we feel stressed, upset, or angry? You guessed it—we turn to our best friend for comfort ... food.

GET PSYCHED

"I teach my children that holidays and special events are more about what we do as a family and less about what we eat." –*Meredith, New Jersey*

Fortunately, the news about holiday weight gain isn't all bad. A study published in the *New England Journal of Medicine* in 2000 reported that Americans tend to gain only a pound during the holidays, far less than the 5- or 10-pound gain commonly believed. The flip side? Researchers said Americans tend not to lose that extra pound during the year. Weight gain over the holidays, thus, compounds from season to season.

You can do a lot to get through holidays and other special events:

Next time you're at a party where there's a lot of food, observe how the slim people around you eat. They may be involved in conversation with another guest, which takes their focus away from food. They may spend a long time nursing a drink or nibbling on their meal, thereby giving their stomachs time to feel satisfied. Use your observations to build a game plan for yourself.

Avoid showing up at events with an empty stomach. Eat a sensible, healthful meal beforehand, and you'll stand a greater chance of sticking to your meal plan.

If you can't avoid the food—for example, a family Thanksgiving dinner—give yourself permission to indulge before you arrive at the event. A small slice of pumpkin pie or some extra turkey won't derail your long-term plans, as long as you get back on your eating plan the next day. You can also make arrangements to cut back on your food or increase your activity level the day before or after the event to make up for the "planned cheat."

Consider telling your hosts about your diet ahead of time. You can say something such as "I'm trying to cut back on saturated fats—will you be serving vegetables or salad?" Or offer to bring a dish of your own if you feel there won't be any safe choices for you at the event.

What makes you put on weight are the habits and behaviors you engage in day after day after day. You can choose to go easy on yourself over the holidays, especially if you know you won't have any trouble getting back to normal when they're over, or adapt your diet to the season. Either way, you can overcome a brief fluctuation in weight with some prior planning and additional effort.

Postpartum Weight Loss

Pregnancy brings relief from dieting for many women. It's one of the only times in your life when you're encouraged to *gain* weight—what a relief! Many women turn to a healthful diet to nurture the child growing inside. Still others figure pregnancy is a time to pig out—after all, when the baby is born, you can lose all the weight, right? Pregnancy is the perfect opportunity to adopt a "play now, pay later" attitude.

But pregnancy weight is a double-edged sword. After baby arrives, there's tremendous societal pressure to lose all the weight you gained during pregnancy—and quickly. What mom hasn't been subject to a comment such as "I lost all my pregnancy weight before I left the hospital"? If you struggle with your weight, comments such as these can put even more pressure—and instill a sense of competitiveness—on dieting. And if you did put on more weight than you should have during pregnancy, the pressure may feel even greater. And because you're no longer pregnant, it can be difficult to cut back on the eating you've gotten used to over the last 9 months.

> ## GET PSYCHED
>
> "After my daughter was born, I had an extra 15 pounds on my body. Everyone told me I looked fine, but I didn't feel fine. Then it hit me one day; I didn't have to accept those extra 15 pounds. I knew then I wasn't doomed to carry the weight the rest of life." –*Meredith, New Jersey*

Even the slimmest, fittest women are shocked by the physical changes pregnancy and childbirth brings. Immediately after birth, your stomach muscles are loose and flabby, your breasts are full and tender, and you probably have extra padding all over your body, especially around your hips and thighs. The extra padding is courtesy of biology; it's there to help nourish the baby during pregnancy and breast-feeding. Moreover, research shows women grow additional fat cells during the last trimester of pregnancy. Unfortunately, fat cells can shrink with weight loss and exercise, but they never completely disappear, which is why many women have a difficult time getting back to their prepregnancy shape.

This doesn't mean you're doomed to carry extra pregnancy weight forever. Your body may have a different shape after pregnancy, but you can still lose weight, get fit, and feel great after a baby.

Experts recommend you not even think about dieting during the first 6 weeks after the baby's birth. For one thing, you're probably wiped out from the stress of childbirth, or surgery if you've had a C-section, and getting used to a new baby takes time. If you're nursing, you need to build up a good supply of milk. Spend those 6 weeks taking care of yourself and baby by eating well, resting, and recovering. Getting fresh air and moderate, gentle exercise can be good for you physically as well as mentally during this transition time.

WEB TALK: Use ParentCenter's postpartum weight-loss calculator at: www.babycenter.com/calculators/postpartumweight/?_requestid=336306

Here are other tips to keep in mind:

- Check with your ob/gyn before embarking on a diet or exercise program. Your body may not have healed enough to begin certain strength-training exercises, or you may have some nutritional or hormonal deficiencies to correct first.

- Don't rush postpartum weight loss. It took you nine months (or more) to put the weight on. You can't expect to lose it in a matter of weeks. Set a reasonable goal, one that works with your new schedule as a mother.

- Get into a routine of walking with your baby. Not only will you burn extra calories with the exercise, but you'll introduce your child to an active lifestyle at the earliest age.

- If you were eating healthily during pregnancy, don't stop! Practice portion control, or eat smaller meals more frequently during the day to keep up your energy.

Breast-Feeding

If you're a new mother, you're probably well versed in all the benefits of breast-feeding. One of the most widely touted benefits is that it helps you lose the weight you gained during pregnancy. You may have also heard that breast-feeding requires you to eat additional calories every day to help you produce enough milk for your baby. Studies show that breast-feeding mothers lose up to 1½ pounds a month during the four to six months postpartum and continue to lose weight after that time as long as they're still nursing. They also tend to lose more weight than mothers who formula-feed their babies—even more than the moms who are dieting.

Yet after several months of nursing—as well as increasing caloric intake—many breast-feeding moms step on the scales and are shocked to see their post-baby weight hasn't budged—or worse, they weigh more than they did when they were pregnant!

Breast-feeding *does* burn an additional 500 to 600 calories a day. And it's also true that nursing mothers need to increase their calories to accommodate the needs of their nursing child. However, the other part of the equation is that these extra calories are on top of the calories you needed each day to maintain your *prepregnancy* weight—not what you weighed during the pregnancy. This is often what stalls weight loss during breast-feeding.

If you're a nursing mother, you shouldn't do any drastic calorie cutting. But if you're not losing weight while breast-feeding, you should look at how much food you're consuming each day. Are you eating a lot of empty calories or eating like you're still pregnant? If you've started weaning, or you supplement with formula, you might not be burning as many calories as you think you are during breast-feeding.

Be sure to keep the following in mind:

- Keep yourself well-hydrated. Thirst is often mistaken for hunger. Also, good hydration keeps up a steady milk supply. Try sipping on a glass of water every time you sit down to nurse.

- Take extra care not to lose too much weight while breast-feeding. Rapid weight loss is associated with diminished milk supply.

- Join a breast-feeding support group. You'll meet other new mothers who are interested in losing weight. Look for a group run by a lactation specialist, registered nurse, or dietician through a local hospital or breast-feeding organization.

- Aim for a nutritious, balanced diet. If you've been nursing for several months and would like to lose weight a little more quickly, reduce calories only slightly and increase your activity level to burn more calories.

Aging

"When I turned 30, I gained 10 pounds overnight." "I have to exercise twice as hard at age 40 to get the same benefits I did at age 20." "Now that I'm 50, I can't get rid of this spare tire around my middle—it won't budge!" Gaining weight as we age is such a common rite of passage, we even have names for it such as "middle-age spread" or "the battle of the bulge."

Age-related weight gain is a tough battle. According to the John Hancock Center for Physical Activity and Nutrition at Tufts University, people over 40 tend to lose anywhere from ⅓ to ½ pound of muscle each year, which gets replaced with the same weight in fat. Loss of muscle translates into a slower metabolism. So if you're eating the same way you've always eaten, you'll start to gain weight because your BMR has slowed.

On top of this, age-related hormonal changes affect fat stores. As women approach and enter menopause, their levels of estrogen decrease, which has the unfortunate effect of distributing fat around the belly area. With men, testosterone levels decrease, which causes them to lose muscle and increase fat. Aging also slows us down physically—we might not feel like exercising as much as we did when we were younger. However, we may still eat the same way we did, so we become overweight and perhaps even obese.

Although we can't stop aging, we still have a lot of power to affect our weight. Weight gain doesn't have to be something we accept. It's a signal we have to stay active and adjust our food intake. We simply don't need as much food as we did when we were younger, and we can get by with eating less. This is a difficult concept for many people to understand, and even more difficult to adopt.

The solution to age-related weight gain is simple: you need to get more active and eat less. If your body is losing muscle mass, it's more important than ever to start exercising and engaging in activities that build muscle. (Yes, build muscle. Your body, no matter if it's 40 or 80, still has the ability to build muscle.) Especially if you're moderately or very active, you can often eat as well, or even better, than you did when you were younger, because let's face it, many of us didn't eat very well in our teens and 20s.

If you stay active, there's no need to give in to the common wisdom that age equals fat. Many people in their 40s, 50s, and 60s say exercise and healthy eating has them in the best shape of their lives!

Plateaus

You've been tracking your food intake, walking two miles every day rain or shine, and losing weight at one pound a week. Suddenly, your weight loss stops, and nothing you do makes the scale budge. Week after week, the number on your scale holds steady. What has gone wrong? Are you incapable of losing any more weight? Why is your body resisting you?

You've hit what dieting experts call a plateau, and before you get even more discouraged, please be assured plateaus are completely normal with weight loss. Here are some of the reasons why they happen:

When you have a lot of weight to lose it's often easier at the beginning of your diet to lose weight. But as you start nearing your goal weight, weight loss slows or stalls for the simple reason that you were reducing more calories with your higher BMR. Now that your BMR is lower, the reduction in calories isn't as great, so weight loss slows or stalls.

You may be weighing yourself at different times in the week. Weight fluctuates from day to day. For example, if you're female, you may weigh more before your period, and the difference can be measured in pounds. Or one week you may weigh yourself on a Tuesday morning and next weigh yourself on Friday after a high-sodium meal and find you've gained. Try weighing yourself once a week under the same conditions, and you may be pleasantly surprised to see your weight loss hasn't stalled at all.

You may be exercising too much—or cutting back on too many calories. Remember the "feast or famine" lesson in Chapter 4. If your body senses it's being starved, it'll do anything to hold on to the weight. If you sense your recent dieting or exercise schedule has gotten too aggressive, back off for a few weeks.

Your body may have gotten bored with your diet and exercise routine. Try shifting nutrients in your diet—if you've been eating low-carb, add some salads or whole grains to your meals over the next few days and see what happens. Or if you're eating too many carbs, cut back. Run a different route over the week, adding hills and hand weights.

If you've been keeping a food diary, examine it to see where your eating habits have changed. Have you been eating more than you previously thought? Have you begun snacking at bedtime or reaching for cookies when you're stressed during the day?

Depression

The link between depression and weight gain is a little like the proverbial chicken and egg. Does gaining weight and becoming overweight make you depressed? Or does depression make you overweight?

Depression is caused by an imbalance of two chemicals in the brain, serotonin and norepinephrine, which are believed to regulate mood as well as reduce feelings of pain throughout the body. Depression can have many causes, and depressive episodes can range from mild to severe. Only a trained medical or mental health doctor can make a diagnosis of depression and prescribe a course of treatment to alleviate symptoms.

Scientists aren't sure which comes first, but the two conditions are inexorably linked. Many people tend not to be happy or feel good about themselves when they're carrying more weight than they want. Other overweight people do battle with chronic self-esteem issues and poor body image, both of which are linked to depression. Another link to depression and weight is through ill health. People who suffer from chronic illness such as heart disease, joint disorders, and diabetes are more apt to develop depression; many of these conditions are brought on through overweight and obesity. Some researchers even suspect dieting can cause depression, especially when a patient gets caught up in a chronic cycle of losing and gaining weight.

WEB TALK: Take a free, confidential depression screening test at:

 www.depression-screening.org

Q&A

I've been taking an antidepressant over the last year. I haven't changed my diet, but I notice I'm beginning to gain weight and it's making me feel worse.

One of the unfortunate side effects of long-term antidepressant use is weight change. Antidepressants can affect weight by increasing or decreasing basic metabolic rate (BMR), or they can cause hormonal changes and affect appetite. Some drugs can even increase cravings for certain types of foods.

Side effects vary among types of antidepressants. Some selective serotonin reuptake inhibitors (SSRIs) may cause everything from increased breast size to carbohydrate cravings. Anticonvulsants prescribed for some mood disorders can cause elevated blood insulin and increased appetite leading to weight gain.

Do *not* stop taking your antidepressants. Make an appointment today to talk to your doctor about your weight and what you can do to control it, as well as your depression.

If your weight is making you depressed—or you suspect depression is making you gain—make an appointment with your physician and/or mental health professional today to discuss your concerns. If you suspect depression is a problem for you, don't try to treat the condition on your own or attempt to "get over it." Depression is an illness that requires professional help.

If you're diagnosed with mild or moderate depression, your doctor should encourage you to exercise. The studies on the benefits of exercise on depression are numerous. In fact, some mild cases of depression respond well to exercise without medication— with the added benefit of burning calories.

Track in your food journal how food affects your mood. You may begin to discern a pattern between your intake of sweets and short-term feelings of depression, for example. Try changing your diet to see if the feelings are alleviated.

If your weight is causing you to feel suicidal, get help immediately. Call 911 or your mental health-care provider, or just get yourself to an emergency room. If this is too much for you, then tell someone you trust how you're feeling so they can get you the care you need.

Eating Disorders

According to published medical literature, there's a strong link between dieting and eating disorders. An eating disorder is a recognized illness, according to the National Institutes of Mental Health; it is not simply a condition brought on through a failure of willpower or behavior.

According to the American Psychological Association, eating disorders exist in three types.

Anorexia nervosa is characterized by a distorted self-image. Someone with this condition sees themselves as "fat," although they're thin—sometimes dangerously so. People with this disorder cut their food to starvation levels, engage in excessive exercising, and often engage in behaviors such as refusing to eat in front of other people. Anorexics often lose large amounts of weight, to the point of serious illness, even death.

WEB TALK: To learn more about eating disorders and how they're treated, visit the National Eating Disorders website at:

www.nationaleatingdisorders.org

Bulimia nervosa is characterized by a cycle of bingeing and purging. Someone with bulimia eats large amounts of food, often in secret, and then purges themselves of the food and feelings of guilt by vomiting, using laxatives, enemas, or diuretics, or through excessive exercise. These purging activities bring them some psychological relief until the next time they binge.

Binge eating disorder is similar to bulimia nervosa, except the binger does not purge the food. Binge eaters frequently engage in episodes of out-of-control eating while dealing with feelings of anger and self-loathing.

Females are more at risk for developing an eating disorder than males; however, an estimated 5 to 15 percent of eating disorder sufferers are male, so it's not a "women's only" disease. Nor is it a condition only affecting young people. Anyone can develop an eating disorder at any age.

Researchers aren't sure why people develop eating disorders, although they do know certain psychological factors predispose people to the illness. These factors include a need for perfection (anorexia) or a history of impulsiveness (bulimia). There is some evidence that environment has a role in the disease. Some sufferers report they were teased by family members about their bodies or weight, which led them to start starving, bingeing, or purging.

Unfortunately, eating disorders are more likely to go untreated than other psychological conditions. If you suspect you're developing a problem with your eating, get help! Although it may be hard, confiding in a family member or close friend can help you deal with what you're going through. If it's easier to talk to a stranger, contact the National Eating Disorders Association's toll-free helpline at 1-800-931-2237. They'll be able to point you to resources near your home.

WEB TALK: Learn more about treatment options for eating disorders at:

www.nationaleatingdisorders.org/p.asp?WebPage_ID=295

It seems like I'm always obsessing about my weight. Could I be at risk for developing an eating disorder?

It's hard to say. The American Psychological Association points out that most people worry about their weight occasionally. Someone with an eating disorder takes that worry to an extreme, engaging in eating behaviors and habits that wreak serious havoc on their health and well-being.

You have to ask yourself how your behaviors and habits affect your daily life. For example, are you constantly telling yourself how fat you are and comparing your body to others? Do you think about your diet to the exclusion of everything else in your life? Are you engaging in behaviors you hide from your friends and family, such as vomiting after meals or hoarding food so you can eat alone? These signs, and more, indicate a talk with a psychologist who specializes in eating disorders is in order.

The bottom line: if you or people close to you are worried about your dieting behavior, then it's a wise idea to talk to a mental health professional or your physician.

What You Can Do

Keep in mind that every dieter—even the most enthusiastic ones—are going to have tough moments that test their commitment to weight loss. You can let those moments derail you, or you can choose to handle them and learn something new—and possibly life-changing—about yourself. Look at these challenges as an opportunity to grow and change every aspect of your life for the better.

☐ Remember that weight loss isn't just about food and exercise; it's also about how you feel. Get in touch with your moods, your reactions to certain events, and how you cope with life. Understanding how you behave can tell you a lot about how you eat.

☐ If you tend to reach for food when you're stressed or bored or angry, remember that this urge is just a habit. You can learn to replace it with another habit, such as reaching for your journal, a knitting project, or even a low-calorie treat.

☐ There's always a solution for a weight-loss challenge. If something feels impossible to you—such as getting through the holiday season without gaining weight—you just haven't considered all your options. Get creative when your diet plans don't mesh with your life, and you'll be surprised at what you can deal with!

☐ If problems relating to your weight loss are too overwhelming for you—for example, you feel depressed or even want to die—get help immediately. Do not try to treat yourself or let someone tell you you can "snap out of it." You need help, and you need it now.

☐ Remember to take it easy on yourself. If you've been losing weight steadily and you're happy with your progress, don't beat yourself up if you go off your diet for a week. One week of lousy eating isn't what made you gain weight—it was a lifetime of lousy eating. Forgive yourself and move on.

Part 4

Beyond the Diet

Congratulations! You're either doing quite well with your plan and losing weight steadily, or you've met your weight-loss goals. In these final chapters, you learn how to cope with other health conditions affecting or influencing weight loss, how to keep up the momentum by finding the right support—and how to give support, too. And you see what life can be like after weight loss.

Doctor's Orders

You've heard the statistics and know that being overweight or obese puts you at risk for all kinds of diseases and disorders. You may have thought, *Well, I'm just a little overweight, so I don't have to worry* or *Yeah, I'm carrying 100 pounds more than I should, but last time I went to the doctor, he said I was healthy as a horse.*

The problem with many health conditions and diseases affected by overweight and obesity is that they sneak up on you. You may find you have high blood pressure, high cholesterol, or type 2 diabetes during a routine doctor's visit or a physical for a new job. Or worse, you might find you have a significant heart disease *after* suffering a major heart attack.

Now you have a new health condition to cope with as well as overweight and obesity. Sometimes you even have two or three additional conditions to contend with, because they all seem to be linked. You may be feeling frightened because this is the first time you've ever been unwell. You're ready to do anything and everything your doctor says to reverse your condition and feel better.

On the other hand, you may be feeling ambivalent. Perhaps your doctor told you you'd better watch your cholesterol because it's borderline high, but you're just not ready to begin eating "rabbit food" for the rest of your life. What are your options?

Combined with the miracles of modern medicine, small health changes you make in your life can reap huge benefits for your overall health, specific health conditions, and quality of life. Some people do so well with diet, exercise, and lifestyle changes alone that they manage to control their health conditions without medications and avoid painful, dangerous surgeries.

When You Must *Lose* Weight

There may come a time when losing weight stops being something you'll do tomorrow and something you must start today. Overweight/obesity is the second leading cause of preventable death in the United States (tobacco is the first). Overweight and obesity increase the risk of heart disease and other health conditions, including high blood pressure, high blood cholesterol, type 2 diabetes, stroke, and a number of cancers. In fact, it's associated with more than 30 medical conditions, and studies have proven its strong relationship with at least 15 of those 30 conditions.

GET PSYCHED

"What you need from your health provider is not a magic bullet but a magical attitude, one of respect for you as a valuable human being."
–*Victoria Moran in* Fit from Within

At some point in your life, perhaps when you're sitting across from your physician listening to your diagnosis, you'll finally understand how overweight or obesity has finally caught up to you. With any luck, you'll be ready to make some changes. Some of them may be surprisingly easy for you to make, such as beginning an exercise program; others may be harder, such as beginning a weight-loss plan, especially if you have a lot of weight to lose.

On a positive note, having a medical trigger that inspires and motivates your weight loss may have a silver lining. Researchers studied three groups of successful dieters in the National Weight Control Registry (NWCR) for the link between medical triggers and weight loss. In an article published in the September 2004 issue of *Preventive Medicine*, one group reported medical triggers that made them lose weight, the second group had nonmedical triggers, and the third said they had no triggers at all. The people who had medical triggers guiding their weight loss reported greater initial weight loss than the other two groups, and they also gained less weight over 2 years.

Dealing With Denial Denial is a common reaction after getting a medical diagnosis, especially if you had no idea anything was wrong. *High blood pressure? Are you sure? But I barely eat salt!* you tell your doctor. Or *I can't have breast cancer. No one in my family has ever had it.* It can take a few days or maybe even weeks for the diagnosis to sink in. When it does, you may feel frightened or angry. You'll probably want to go for a second opinion, and that's encouraged.

> **GET PSYCHED**
>
> "Blame is demeaning; responsibility is empowering." *–Victoria Moran in* Fit from Within

After you've accepted your condition, the denial wears off. This can happen a few ways. You may begin a course of therapy that has you feeling better than you've felt in a long time. You may have searched the Internet and found support groups of other people with the same condition you have and realized your life isn't over. It simply may be that you needed time to accept that things are different for you now.

We've all heard about diehard smokers who, after being diagnosed with cancer, continue to smoke, sometimes going as far as taking puffs through their tracheotomies. This is denial pushed to its most extreme form. If you can't seem to move beyond the denial stage, here's what you can do:

- Write a letter to yourself, or write in your journal. What are you feeling? Angry? Blasé? Cheated? What bothers you most about your diagnosis?

- Talk to a trusted friend or family member. Ask them what they think you're avoiding. Sometimes others can clearly see what we fail to see in ourselves.

- Be honest with your health-care professionals. Let them know how you're feeling. They may have some valuable insight into your condition and assure you that many of their other patients feel the same way.

Be kind to yourself. Facing a major health crisis is not the time for blame and recriminations. Focus on understanding your condition and moving past the denial.

Overcoming Resistance Resistance is another normal human tendency. Sometimes we know we have to do something—make a difficult phone call, for example—but we can't seem to pick up the phone. We often even resist doing the things we know are good for us, such as eating our 5 to 8 servings of vegetables per day or flossing after meals.

But when you're facing a serious health crisis, resistance can be bad for you—even kill you. Resistance can take many forms, including the following:

- Not monitoring your blood glucose levels as closely as you should

- Eating the foods that contributed to you developing the condition
- Keeping up habits such as cigarette smoking, excessive alcohol consumption, and a sedentary lifestyle
- Skipping medication and doctor appointments

If you're feeling resistance to making changes, the ways to get around it are similar to the ways you got around denial. Ask yourself *Why am I resisting quitting smoking?* In this case, your answer may be, *Because it's hard. Because I love to smoke. I've smoked for 40 years, and I don't think I can ever give it up. Plus, whenever I've quit smoking, I've gained weight.*

Bring those answers to your caregiver. What suggestions can she make to help you overcome those objections? Perhaps she can make quitting easier for you by prescribing a medication such as Wellbutrin. She may also tell you that gaining a few pounds might not be terrible for you while you're quitting, or point out there's a very successful smoking-cessation group at your local hospital that has achieved good results with hard-core smokers.

Cardiovascular Diseases

Heart disease and stroke account for more than 40 percent of all deaths in the United States each year, with heart disease being the number one cause of death and stroke being number three. One death every 33 seconds can be attributed to cardiovascular disease. Once thought to be a disease of men and older people, cardiovascular disease is proving to be a major killer of women and people in their 30s and 40s. Currently, one fourth of the U.S. population suffers from some form of cardiovascular disease.

PsychSpeak

Lipids are fatty substances found in the bloodstream and body tissues. Cholesterol and triglycerides are considered lipids.

And the kicker? Cardiovascular disease is one of the most preventable diseases of all the serious diseases affecting Americans today. Overweight and obesity increase the risk of illness and death from coronary artery disease (CAD), for example, because of associated high blood *lipid* levels. And because the disease develops over time, overweight and obese children run the risk of developing CAD later in life.

Yet study after study shows your risk of developing cardiovascular disease can be significantly reduced through a proper diet, regular exercise, and other moderate lifestyle changes. As little as a 5 to 10 percent weight loss can reduce total blood cholesterol—a major factor in the development of heart disease.

Mark B. Davidson, a Westford, Massachusetts–based physician, recommends that dieters who have heart disease or a family his-

you're not alone

Ten or fifteen years ago, my physician told me I had a heart murmur, so I was sent to a cardiologist for a checkup. She said one of my valves was blocked, and at some point I would need surgery.

I decided at that point to cut out fats from my diet. No cheese, no good stuff. I can't remember if my doctor recommended that I do this, but I did it. And I started walking around my neighborhood. I took it slow at first, maybe 10 minutes a day, and built on that. One day I took the car out and traced my route, and it was 2 miles. By cutting out fat and walking, I lost 51 pounds.

The hills on the route got to be too much for me, so I started walking in my basement. I listened to books on tape from the library. Each tape is 45 minutes on each side, so

tory of heart disease first schedule an appointment with their family physician for a thorough checkup. The patient and the doctor can identify and discuss different risk factors that might make certain types of weight-loss plans more risky based on the patient's health history and current health. During the appointment, your physician can also give you an idea of initial weight-loss goals and your ideal weight based on a loose interpretation of the body mass index (BMI) and/or height and weight tables. Davidson also points out that a complete physical can identify other causes of obesity, such as hypothyroidism.

During this appointment, you should be prepared to discuss other significant health factors you have, such as diabetes, smoking, a history of early-onset CVD in your family, high cholesterol (especially unusually high LDL or low HDL cholesterol numbers), high triglycerides, a sedentary lifestyle, or a previous history of CAD.

I'd walk that long. Having a good book to listen to made a big difference— I couldn't wait to go to the basement. But when the book was boring, it wasn't fun.

The lowest weight I got to was 122 pounds. People thought I was too thin. Eventually I added more fat to my diet, and along with my reduced walking, I ended up gaining 25 pounds back. I would like to weigh 135 pounds; that's a good weight for me. Up until recently, I was working out at Curves with my daughter, but then I broke both wrists when I fell during a vacation. I hope I'll be able to get back to exercising when I'm healed.

—Jane, 77, Hartford, Connecticut

High Blood Cholesterol High blood cholesterol presents no symptoms, so to determine if you have it, you must have a blood test that measures the levels of LDL (bad) cholesterol, HDL (good) cholesterol, and triglycerides in your bloodstream. Your diagnosis may come as a complete surprise to you. Your doctor will probably tell you that having high blood cholesterol puts you at risk for a number of diseases, especially heart disease.

Cholesterol is a fatty substance found in every cell of the human body. It actually helps our bodies make hormones and certain substances that help us digest food. Our bodies produce cholesterol, and we also get it from the foods we eat. Some people naturally produce high amounts of cholesterol while others produce very little. Most people produce just enough and manage to keep their cholesterol levels stable with a proper diet.

Over time, high blood cholesterol can wreak havoc throughout your body. It begins to stick to the walls of your arteries, creating buildup called plaque. When too much plaque builds up, several things can happen. If it builds up in arteries throughout the body, it causes a condition called atherosclerosis, or hardening of the arteries (more on that later in this chapter). If it builds up in the coronary arteries, which bring blood to your heart, it can develop into coronary artery disease. With this condition, blood flow and oxygen to the heart is decreased. The lack of blood flow to the heart muscle can cause immense pain, called angina. Other times, soft plaque in the arteries can break off the artery walls and enter the bloodstream, causing clots that block or partially block arteries. The organ supplied by the blocked artery doesn't get blood and oxygen, so the organ's cells become severely damaged, and in some cases, die.

Your doctor will determine if you have high blood cholesterol by comparing your numbers to a chart similar to the following one. Cholesterol levels are measured in milligrams (mg) of cholesterol per deciliter (dL) of blood.

Total Cholesterol Level	Total Cholesterol Category
Less than 200mg/dL	Desirable
200 to 239mg/dL	Borderline high
240mg/dL and above	High

LDL Cholesterol Level	LDL Cholesterol Category
Less than 100mg/dL	Optimal
100 to 129mg/dL	Near optimal/above optimal
130 to 159mg/dL	Borderline high
160 to 189mg/dL	High
190mg/dL and above	Very high

HDL Cholesterol Level	HDL Cholesterol Category
Less than 40mg/dL	A major risk factor for heart disease
40 to 59mg/dL	The higher, the better
60mg/dL and above	Considered protective against heart disease

From the National Institute of Health's National Heart, Blood, and Lung Institute.

Your doctor will also look at your triglycerides number. *Triglycerides*, like cholesterol, are fatty substances in your bloodstream. High triglycerides can also raise your risk for heart disease. Levels that are borderline high (150 to 199mg/dL) or high (200mg/dL or more) may need treatment, depending on your risk factors for heart disease.

When you get a diagnosis of high blood cholesterol, your doctor will recommend that you make some changes. Sometimes

PsychSpeak

Triglycerides are fatty substances that are a stored form of energy in the blood. Elevated triglyceride levels may be caused by food or alcohol and can signal a risk for heart disease.

the changes are minor; other times, depending on your other risk factors for heart disease, the changes are sweeping. The most commonly suggested changes include the following:

- Eating a diet low in cholesterol and saturated fat and high in soluble fiber—such as oats, beans, and apples. Your doctor may also ask you to switch to cholesterol-lowering margarines.
- Beginning an exercise program if you haven't started one. Regular exercise has been proven to lower LDL cholesterol and raise HDL cholesterol.
- Losing weight if you are overweight or obese, especially if you have high blood cholesterol with high triglycerides, low HDL cholesterol, and a large waist measurement (more than 40 inches for men and 35 inches for women).
- Taking cholesterol-lowering drugs.

Drug treatment controls but does not "cure" high blood cholesterol, so it's important to make the appropriate dietary and activity level changes in your life as well. On the other hand, if your doctor does prescribe medication, you should not discontinue taking it if you feel you can control your cholesterol through diet and exercise alone. In some cases, diet and exercise are not enough to bring cholesterol levels to normal levels.

High Blood Pressure As with high blood cholesterol, high blood pressure is a condition that doesn't present any symptoms. It's often called "the silent killer," and with good reason: uncontrolled, it can lead to stroke, heart failure, heart attack, kidney failure, and blindness. It's a condition more likely to affect African Americans, which accounts for the higher rates of heart disease they suffer. More than half of everyone over age 60 has high blood pressure, and 75 percent of high blood pressure cases are directly attributable to overweight and obesity. Your chance of developing high blood pressure is 5 to 6 times more likely if you're obese and between the ages of 20 to 45 than it is if you're a healthy weight for your age and body type.

Blood pressure is simply the measure of the force of the blood against your arterial walls. The force in the arteries when the heart beats is called systolic pressure, and the force when it's at rest is called diastolic pressure. Both are measured in millimeters of mercury (mm Hg).

The systolic and diastolic pressure numbers are presented together in a sort of fraction: your systolic pressure appears over your diastolic pressure. Your doctor will be looking for a number that is lower than 120/80. At 140/90 or higher, you have high blood pressure, although in people with chronic kidney disease or diabetes, blood pressure of 130/80 is considered high blood pressure. If you're right on the border of either of these numbers, your doctor will certainly recommend some lifestyle and dietary changes. These may include the following:

Eating a healthy diet. Clinical studies show a diet that emphasized fruits, vegetables, and low-fat dairy foods and one that was low in saturated fats, total fats, and cholesterol reduced blood pressure. A diet based on this study, called DASH, which stands for "Dietary Approaches to Stop Hypertension," was developed by the National Heart, Lung, and Blood Institute. Details can be found at nhlbi.nih.gov/health/public/heart/hbp/dash/index.htm.

Reducing dietary salt and sodium. There's sodium in just about everything you eat, from bread and milk to vegetables and even fruit. Low sodium in the diet keeps blood pressure from rising and helps prescribed medications work better.

Maintaining a healthy weight. Blood pressure rises as body weight increases. Losing 10 pounds can lower blood pressure.

Exercising. It plays a major role in reducing your chances of developing heart disease.

Limiting alcohol. Alcohol raises blood pressure.

Quitting smoking. Smoking hastens the damaging effects of high blood pressure because it injures blood vessel walls and contributes to hardening of the arteries.

Taking blood pressure medication and self-monitoring blood pressure at home.

The key with blood pressure is to catch it early and treat it quickly before it escalates into other problems. With the right management plan, you can control your high blood pressure, as well as your weight, and lead a long, healthy life.

Atherosclerosis Atherosclerosis is a slow, stealthy disease that often starts in childhood, culminating in serious heart disease later in life. Commonly called "hardening of the arteries," atherosclerosis is when arteries throughout the body harden and narrow due to the buildup of plaque. It can affect arteries in the brain, kidneys, arms, and legs, as well as in the heart (coronary artery disease; more on this later in this chapter). You probably won't exhibit any symptoms of atherosclerosis until the artery (or arteries) affected is partially and/or totally blocked.

Arteries affected by atherosclerosis get blocked with either hard or soft plaque. If the plaque is hard, it can cause arteries to get thick and stiff; the soft plaque is liable to break up and enter the blood stream, causing a blood clot. Then the blood clot can partially or totally block the flow of blood into the organ supplied by the artery. If that organ is your brain, you will suffer a stroke. If it's your heart, you'll experience a heart attack.

When you're diagnosed with atherosclerosis, your doctor will probably recommend you ...

- Eat a healthy diet low in fats, cholesterol, and sodium, and consume plenty of fruits, vegetables, and low-fat dairy.
- Refrain from smoking.
- Begin an exercise program, if you haven't started one already.
- Lose weight, if you're overweight or obese.

Your doctor may prescribe medications that lower your cholesterol and blood pressure if they're high. You may also be prescribed anticoagulants to prevent blood clots from forming. Moreover, your doctor may recommend aspirin therapy, which has been shown to prevent blood platelets from clumping to form clots.

With serious blockages, surgery may be required. Some common surgeries for atherosclerosis include ...

- Angioplasty.
- Coronary artery bypass surgery.
- Carotid artery surgery.
- Bypass surgery of the leg arteries.

Angioplasty opens blocked or narrowed coronary arteries. It can improve the blood flow to your heart, relieve chest pain, and possibly prevent a heart attack. Sometimes a small metal coil or mesh tube called a stent is placed in the artery to keep it open after the procedure.

During coronary artery bypass surgery, arteries or veins from other areas in your body are used to bypass the blocked coronary arteries. This surgery can improve blood flow to your heart, relieve chest pain, and possibly prevent a heart attack.

In carotid artery surgery, plaque buildup from the carotid artery in the neck is removed, improving blood flow to the brain.

With bypass surgery of the leg arteries, a healthy blood vessel is used to bypass the narrowed or blocked blood vessels. The healthy blood vessel redirects blood around the blocked artery, improving blood flow to the leg.

These surgical procedures are major surgeries. You'll probably want to do everything you can before resorting to surgery. Fortunately, lifestyle changes can improve many of the symptoms of atherosclerosis.

Coronary Artery Disease Coronary artery disease (CAD) is a condition that results from atherosclerosis, or hardening of the arteries. Half a million Americans die each year from CAD, which makes it the number one killer of both men and women of all heart diseases. Undiagnosed and untreated CAD often leads to heart attacks—many of them fatal. Some risk factors for CAD cannot be controlled, but a great many of them can be bettered through diet, exercise, and other lifestyle changes.

A diagnosis of CAD means blood isn't getting to your heart because the arteries that supply it are narrowing and hardening due to a buildup of plaque. When oxygen and blood don't get to your heart, you can have a heart attack. Unlike high blood pressure or high cholesterol, you may have noticed some signs of CAD, such as pain that may have brought you to your doctor. The pain, called angina, is caused by lack of oxygen to the heart muscle. When the plaque is soft, it can dislodge and enter the bloodstream. Your blood responds by clotting, and sometimes the clots can lead to the pain of a heart attack, although *it's important to note that some heart attacks cause minor or no pain at all.*

If you're suffering from CAD, your doctor may ask you to ...

- Adopt a healthy diet to prevent or reduce high blood pressure and high blood cholesterol and maintain a healthy weight.
- Quit smoking, if you smoke.
- Begin an exercise program, if you don't already exercise.
- Lose weight, if you are overweight or obese.
- Work on reducing your stress.

Your doctor may also prescribe medications that reduce stress on your heart and diminish your chance of suffering a heart attack. Medicines may also prevent or delay major heart surgeries, such as angioplasty or bypass surgery (see the earlier "Atherosclerosis" section).

Heart Attack Every year, 1 million Americans suffer heart attacks, and about half of them die. Half of the people who die pass away in the first hour after the attack, before they get to the hospital. This is because a heart attack often causes arrhythmias that severely decrease the heart's ability to pump blood. Unfortunately, many victims wait hours before seeking treatment, which can result in death or irreparable damage to their hearts.

A heart attack occurs when blood and oxygen to the heart gets blocked, usually by a blood clot, damaging cells and tissue. Most people experience symptoms including chest pain that may also spread to the back, shoulders, arms, neck, or jaw. Other symptoms include shortness of breath, nausea, sweating, or dizziness. Symptoms vary, however, and some people never have any symptoms.

It is imperative that you know the signs of a heart attack so you can act fast to get treatment. Call 911 immediately if you or someone near you exhibits the symptoms of a heart attack.

When you're treated for a heart attack, your doctors work to restore proper blood flow to your heart, monitor your vital signs, and determine what kind of damage the attack has done to your heart. After you're released from medical care, you will be put on a treatment plan that may include cardiac rehab, follow-up visits to your doctors, medications, and lifestyle changes. Most people, after they've suffered a heart attack, can go back to their "normal activities"—driving, work, sex, and travel, for example. Your doctor will likely discourage you from undertaking any "normal activities" that might set you up for another heart attack, such as eating a poor diet and living a sedentary lifestyle.

If your doctor sends you to cardiac rehab, you'll work with doctors, nurses, exercise specialists, dieticians, physical therapists, and/or psychologists to learn how to exercise safely and improve your stamina, as well as understand your heart condition. They'll show you a variety of ways to reduce your risk of future heart problems. Your cardiac rehab team will teach you the skills you need to cope with the stress of adjusting to a new lifestyle.

WEB TALK: Learn all the signs of heart attack, stroke, and cardiac arrest at the American Heart Association:

www.americanheart.org/presenter.jhtml?identifier=3053#Heart_Attack

After a heart attack, most people take daily medications, such as aspirin therapy to keep blood thin, medications that lower cholesterol and/or blood pressure, or other medications that reduce the heart's workload

Many people find that a heart attack is a major wakeup call. Because they've come so close to dying, they're motivated to finally listen to their health-care professional's recommendations about losing weight, exercising more, and adopting a healthier lifestyle. It's a difficult way to get the message, but it's certainly better than not getting a chance to hear it at all.

Type 2 Diabetes

Type 2 diabetes along with overweight and obesity go hand-in-hand. Researchers estimate as many as 90 percent of people with type 2 diabetes are also overweight or obese. When researchers have tried to pinpoint the common variable among people with type 2 diabetes, obesity always comes out on top as the major environmental influence on the disease. Carrying around extra weight makes the disease worse because it increases insulin resistance and glucose intolerance.

Type 2 diabetes is caused when the cells in the muscles, liver, and fat cannot use insulin properly. Over time, the pancreas is unable to make enough insulin for the body's needs. As a result, blood glucose levels increase and the cells don't get the energy they need to work properly. Without treatment, high blood glucose can damage nerves and blood vessels, causing complications such as heart disease, stroke, blindness, kidney disease, nerve problems, gum infections, and amputation.

It's estimated that more than 5 million people in the United States have type 2 diabetes but don't know it, often because people show no signs or symptoms of diabetes. Often their symptoms are so mild that they might not notice them, or they confuse them with other symptoms of overweight and/or obesity—such as hunger or weight loss if they're dieting.

If you're overweight or obese and have any of the following symptoms, talk to your health-care professional:

- Increased thirst
- Increased hunger
- Fatigue
- Increased urination, especially at night
- Weight loss
- Blurred vision
- Sores that do not heal

With early diagnosis of diabetes, damage from the disease can be prevented and the condition itself can be controlled.

Your doctor can use several tests to diagnose type 2 diabetes. The Fasting Plasma Glucose (FPG) is often preferred because it can be done in the morning after an 8-hour fast at night. A fasting glucose level of 100 to 125 mg/dL is called impaired fasting glucose, and it can indicate pre-diabetes. A fasting glucose level of 126 and above indicates diabetes. Normal fasting blood sugar is considered under 99 mg/dL. Some conditions can temporarily make blood sugar numbers higher, such as illness and medication, so when making a diagnosis, your doctor will also consider any symptoms you have, as well as your current health and health history.

WEB TALK: The American Diabetes Association offers live Q&A sessions on its website:

www.diabetes.org/adalive/default.jsp

When you've received a diagnosis of type 2 diabetes, or your doctor suspects you're on your way to developing the disease, you'll be put on a diabetes management plan that is comprised of the following.

Because the link between diabetes and overweight/obesity is so strong, one of the first things your doctor will want you to do is lose weight. A 10 percent reduction in weight can often bring some profound health benefits; studies show even a 5 to 7 percent weight loss can prevent some people from developing the disease.

Make wise food choices to manage your disease. Eating low-fat meals high in fruits, vegetables, and whole grains, and reducing simple carbohydrates and limiting alcohol are common recommendations.

Get physically active. All it takes is 30 minutes a day, 5 days a week. The benefits of exercise for people who are living with type 2 diabetes are truly amazing.

Manage your blood glucose levels through diet and by testing your blood sugar levels throughout the day as indicated by your M.D.

Take all your prescribed medications. It is vitally important that you do not attempt to treat diabetes on your own through food and diet. Do not discontinue taking any medication until you've checked with your physician.

Practice good body care. People with type 2 diabetes are prone to problems with their skin, gums, eyes, and feet, some of which can lead to serious complications, such as infection, blindness, and amputations.

If you smoke, quit.

WEB TALK: Learn about the benefits of weight loss and exercise at the American Diabetes Association's website:

www.diabetes.org/weightloss-and-exercise.jsp

WEB TALK: Download Joslin Diabetes Center's new nutritional and activity guidelines for the overweight and obese at:

https://diabetesmanagement.joslin.org/ Guidelines/Nutrition_ClinGuide.pdf

Studies have shown that having type 2 diabetes raises your risk for depression and other mental health disorders, so learn to recognize the signs of these conditions and report them to your health-care provider. To learn more about the link between depression and type 2 diabetes, visit www.diabetes.org/type-2-diabetes/ depression. jsp.

Cancers

Few words strike as much fear in people as the word *cancer*. When you get that diagnosis, your life is often turned upside down and inside out. Your life as you knew it is never the same.

Cancer affects dozens of organs and body parts, and many kinds of cancers are linked to overweight and obesity, including ...

- Breast Cancer.
- Esophagus and gastric cardia cancers.
- Colorectal cancer.
- Endometrial cancer.
- Renal cell cancer.

Breast cancer. The links between breast cancer and overweight/obesity are startling. Postmenopausal women who are obese have a higher risk of developing breast cancer, and weight gain after menopause may also increase the risk of developing breast cancer. Women who gain 45 pounds or more after age 18 are twice as likely to develop breast cancer after menopause as those who keep a stable weight. Overweight menopausal women aren't the only vulnerable people; premenopausal women diagnosed with breast cancer and who are overweight appear to have a shorter life span than women with a lower BMI. Men also run a higher risk of developing breast cancer when they're obese.

Esophagus and gastric cardia cancers. Obesity is strongly associated with cancer of the esophagus, and the risk becomes higher when the BMI is higher. Moreover, the risk for gastric cardia cancer rises moderately as the BMI is increased.

Colorectal cancer. High BMI, high calorie intake, and low physical activity are all associated with colorectal cancer. A large waist circumference also puts men and women at risk.

Endometrial cancer. Women who are obese have three to four times the risk of endometrial cancer than women with lower BMIs. Obese women with diabetes may have three times the risk for endometrial cancer than those who are obese alone.

Renal cell cancer. Obesity is linked to renal cell (kidney) cancer, especially in women. In one study, overweight was linked to 21 percent of renal cancer cases.

After a cancer diagnosis, you'll get a treatment plan that covers what kind of chemotherapy, radiation therapy, or surgery is appropriate for your disease. Your health-care professional may also ask you to make one or more of these lifestyle changes:

- Eat a diet rich in fruits, vegetables, grains, and fiber.
- Begin an exercise plan before starting any chemotherapy treatments.
- Engage in moderately intense physical activity such as brisk walking or swimming 3 or 4 times each week. Sessions should last between 15 minutes and 1 hour. Longer than that, and you may run the risk of becoming more fatigued.

  If you're extremely fatigued after treatment, don't exercise for a few days. And if exercise worsens your fatigue during treatment, don't exercise.
- Quit smoking.

One condition you'll want to watch out for when you're fighting cancer is neutropenia, which is a common side effect of chemotherapy and immunosuppressive medications. A person can become neutropenic when his or her white blood cells are temporarily reduced to very low levels. A low white blood cell count reduces a person's immune response and makes him susceptible to infection. It's important for neutropenic patients to practice good hygiene, food safety, and sanitation practices, such as frequent hand washing and following a neutropenic or low-bacteria diet. Your doctor may want you to avoid raw salads and fresh fruits when you're neutropenic, as these foods can carry pathogens that lead to infection. A registered dietitian can work with you to develop a low-bacteria diet.

It's important to remember that changing your diet after you've received a cancer diagnosis will not cure the disease. However, improving your diet and making appropriate lifestyle changes can make a huge difference in your quality of life during and after treatment.

WEB TALK: Learn more about complementary and alternative medical practices at the National Institutes of Health–sponsored website: nccam.nih.gov/

Arthritis

In the United States alone, 21 million people suffer the effects of arthritis, and it's one of the leading causes of disability in this country.

Obesity is associated with the development of a form of arthritis called *osteoarthritis* in the hands, the hips, the back, and especially the knees. When your BMI is greater than 25, the likelihood of developing osteoarthritis increases steadily. However, a mere 10- to 15-pound weight loss can relieve symptoms and delay disease progression of osteoarthritis, especially in the knees.

When you're diagnosed with osteoarthritis, your physician may suggest the following:

- Participation in physical/occupational therapy to improve motility and range of motion.
- Weight loss to prevent extra stress on weight-bearing joints.

- Getting your daily requirements of vitamins C, D, and E, which may protect against knee osteoarthritis progression. This is particularly true for vitamin C.

- Strength and endurance exercise programs that help you regain or maintain motion and flexibility.

- Ice or heat treatments.

- Supportive devices such as canes, crutches, walkers, or splints, as well as shock-absorbing footwear and other cushioning devices.

- Complementary and alternative therapies, including nutritional supplements such as glucosamine and chondroitin sulfate.

- Surgery to replace the damaged joint when pain cannot be controlled or eliminated.

PsychSpeak

Osteoarthritis is a degenerative joint disease characterized by a breakdown of the cartilage covering the ends of the bones in a joint. When the cartilage breaks down, the bones rub against each other, resulting in pain and reduced motility. Over time, the joint can become misshapen, and painful bone spurs can grow on the edges of the joint. Moreover, pieces of bone or cartilage can break off and float inside the joint, causing additional pain.

Surgery is obviously the last resort for suffers of osteoarthritis. The good news is that moderate weight loss, along with some easy diet and exercise changes, can vastly improve motility and pain.

Tips on Making—and Sticking With—Changes

Making big changes in your life is hard, especially when you're in the midst of a health crisis. However, the rules for change don't differ much from the rules you'd follow when making changes without a health crisis:

1. Make a plan to change behavior. Write this down.

2. Decide exactly what you will do and when you will do it. For example, if your plan is to lose 20 pounds, you might plan to walk 3 times a week for 20 minutes a day and cut saturated fats from your diet.

3. Plan what you need to get ready. Want to walk? You'll need supportive walking shoes, workout wear, and a place to do your exercise.

4. Think about what might prevent you from reaching your goals. Figure out how you will work around roadblocks.

5. Develop your own cheering section. Who will be there to support you and rally you when you're down?

6. Don't forget those rewards! Especially now, when you make your goals, you'll really want to celebrate your hard work.

You don't have to make big, sweeping changes when you've received a major medical diagnosis. In fact, in many cases it's okay to start slowly. The most important thing to remember is to take any medications or therapies your doctor prescribes. She may even be able to prioritize for you what's most important to change at first. For example, if it's most important for you to control your blood sugar, she may ask you to make dietary changes first before you tackle exercise. After you have your blood sugar under control, then you can move on to developing an exercise routine. In other cases, your doctor may feel your weight is secondary to quitting smoking.

The good news about taking small steps is that one change usually leads right into another. For example, if you're focusing on stabilizing your blood sugar, you may find that you're losing weight with the dietary changes you're making to control those numbers. The weight loss may even stabilize another condition you have, such as high blood pressure. One small change can snowball into one big health turnaround.

My doctor told me I should aim to lose 10 percent of my current body weight. That doesn't seem like much—in fact, I'd still be overweight. What benefit is there to losing such a small amount?

"This statement by your M.D. could mean several things. First, he may be saying that you are slightly overweight and all you need is to increase your exercise and control your portion sizes to bring your weight into the average range. Still, you must remember some people, such as bodybuilders or football players, may never be 'average' weight—they are technically 'overweight' by the numbers, but not necessarily 'overfat.' Body mass index (BMI) and height-weight scales are simply guides, and in some cases, weight can fall a few pounds on either side of their normal ranges based on body frame and other health characteristics without any negative consequences. That's a determination your doctor can make.

"The other point of losing just 10 percent of your weight may be that losing a minimal amount will help you avoid 'yo-yo' dieting, especially if you have a tendency to lose weight quickly, then gain it all back and then some. Losing and maintaining a 10 percent weight loss is easier for a lot of people to grasp. When you've achieved that goal, you can then work on exercise and/or portion control to lose additional weight. Moreover, health conditions such as hypertension and diabetes can be greatly improved by a 10 percent drop in weight—important if your doctor wants to stabilize those conditions in your case.

"My focus, if I were your doctor, would not be solely on the losing of the weight, but rather on how you change your lifestyle to attain and maintain that weight. A 10 percent weight loss will go far in educating you how and why you eat, from sustenance properties and satiety signals, to the emotional and social pulls of food." *—Mark B. Davidson, M.D., a Westford, Massachusetts–based physician associated with Emerson Hospital, Concord, Massachusetts*

What You Can Do

Getting a diagnosis of heart disease, diabetes, or cancer can be one of the scariest events in your life. Once you've accepted that you have this condition, rejoice that you have some options at turning your health around.

- ☐ Learn all you can about your health condition from your health-care professional, trusted Internet sources, and literature.

- ☐ Get a clear treatment plan that prioritizes the changes you need to make in your life.

- ☐ Even though your diagnosis may be frightening or depressing, try to view the situation as an opportunity to turn your health around. Many people with a grim health prognosis manage to make "miraculous" recoveries by simply taking better care of themselves.

- ☐ Always take your medications as directed. Do not try to "cure" yourself or wean yourself off medication on your own. Check with your M.D. before discontinuing any treatment plan.

- ☐ Join a support group for people who share your health challenges. You will probably find other people who are going through the same feelings and treatments you are.

- ☐ Learn to recognize the signs of depression. If you can't shake a lingering case of the blues or you feel your situation is hopeless, get help today.

Getting the Support You Need

Several months have passed—you've said good-bye to 20, 30, maybe even 50 pounds with your eating plan. You've established an exercise routine that's become habit, much to your surprise and delight. Your once-tight clothing fits your leaner form—you've even sprung for some smaller-sized clothing to replace the "fat day" duds you used to depend on. Everyone you know comments on your weight loss—from your boss, who commends you on your perseverance, to your mother, who nags you to eat your favorite chocolate pecan pie she baked especially for you. "You're turning into skin and bones!" she says cheerfully.

And there's the rub. Most of the people who know and care about you will be thrilled that you're taking off pounds and keeping them off. But on your weight-loss journey, you might feel lonely. It could be that your friends and family have never struggled with their weight so they don't know how to support you. It would be great if you could find someone to talk to, someone who really understands how hard dieting is—from staying motivated for months on end to realizing how much it hurts to pass up Mom's pie.

Knowing you can turn to family members, friends, and even strangers when you're battling temptation or stress can make an appreciable difference on your quality of life during a weight-loss program and far beyond. It's simple: the more support you receive, the more likely you are to stick to your diet and keep the lost pounds off.

Everyone Needs Support

Research shows an essential component of successful weight loss includes some kind of ongoing support. Whether informal, such as a husband or friend who tirelessly cheers you on, or formal, such as a hospital-based group meeting, a strong, reliable support system is critical for long-term behavioral change.

The National Self-Help Clearinghouse, a nonprofit organization affiliated with the Graduate School and University Center of the City University of New York, estimates that more than 20 million Americans participate in formal self-help support groups for everything from mental illness and bereavement to disabilities and addictions. On top of those numbers, you have the people who get their support outside of formal programs: from family members and friends who've struggled with similar problems and challenges, to co-workers and strangers in cyberspace who may not know you as well, but who can understand what you're thinking and feeling.

Just as there are dieters in every size, shape, age, color, and sex, there is formal support for those dieters and their specific weight-loss challenges. Do you have more than 100 pounds to lose? There are programs tailor-made for your special needs as a long-term dieter. Are you thinking about bariatric surgery?

Hospitals and universities are rife with support groups for people considering medical options. Can't stop thinking and obsessing about food? Overeaters Anonymous welcomes men, women, and teens who struggle with the emotional side of eating.

One reason formal support programs work so well for dieters is the element of *peer-led support*. Sometimes the program's leader is a former dieter, someone who has lost weight and kept it off, or group leaders can be trained medical or nutritional personnel, too. Nonetheless, the group itself consists of dieters—peers—who are all in the same boat. A group that works well provides members with tools and strategies they may not be able to find elsewhere. It can provide members with structure and accountability, which can lead dieters to persist with an often-difficult lifestyle change. If the meeting is fee-based, that financial element can motivate members.

Peer support doesn't have to come from formal meetings. As a dieter, you have dozens of means and ways to get the help you need.

PsychSpeak

Peer-led support groups are led by people who are actively working on or have succeeded with long-term weight loss. Group leaders usually aren't professionals, although they may be trained in group facilitation and nutrition if they're affiliated with a commercial weight-loss program.

Building Your Personal Support Team

If there's a bright spot in the statistics about the millions of Americans who've dieted or who are dieting now, it's that chances are, dozens of people around you have gone through or are experiencing the physical and mental challenges associated with losing weight. Dieters are a relatively lucky group of people in this respect. Not only do they have a large pool of human support sources to wade through, there's very little stigma attached to dieters and dieting. A person who has a rare medical condition may have to look far and wide for the specialized support he needs and may even have to inquire discreetly to avoid prejudice, judgment, and social estrangement. It's the opposite for a dieter. Because there are so many support resources out in the open, the problem is often how to sort and choose for the best fit. And if you admit to people you're on a diet, it's a good bet they'll start telling you all about their diets!

Even if the people closest to you have never been on a diet, they can still provide valuable support, advice, and inspiration. Barb F., a Weight Watchers group leader and lifetime member from Louisville, Kentucky, points out that although these people may never have struggled with their weight, they often know what you have to do to succeed, and they can push you when you need it the most.

Here are some of the qualities to look for when you're building your personal support team:

- Enthusiasm. You want someone who can celebrate your victories and help you drum up your internal resources when dieting gets tough. Wet blankets need not apply.

- Experience. A person who's walking the same path you are probably has the questions, feelings, or challenges you have. And if they've already walked down the path, they can keep you on the straight and narrow by sharing the wisdom they gained during their experience with weight loss.

- Honesty. "You need people who will tell you what you need to do to get past an urge or a craving," says Barb F. Someone who tells you what you want to hear—who rationalizes why it's okay to give into urges or cravings—is not being honest, but enabling.

- Knowledge. Some people around you eat healthily, exercise, and know exactly what they have to do to stay fit and slim for life. These are people you should watch and listen to; they probably have habits and behaviors you can adopt as you lose weight. Also in this category are the doctors, nutritionists, and fitness experts in your life.

- Compassion. You're going to have days where everything seems to go wrong: you're stressed-out over work, a family member gets sick, you give into an urge and blow your eating plan. Sometimes it's nice to have someone you can lean on, an ear to listen to your woes. Just be sure these are people who can listen while gently nudging you back toward your goals.

Family Your immediate family can be an important source of emotional support while you diet. The people around you are attuned to your behavior and emotions, especially if they live with you, and they can be the first people you turn to when temptation is high and resistance runs low. If you find it difficult to do your weekly food marketing alone, your partner can be enlisted to take over that task for you … or at least accompany you so you don't fill your cart with unhealthy food choices. Children, spouses, and parents can join in with a walk around the block after dinner. The exercise is great for all of you, and a regularly scheduled period of activity brings you together as a family, important when competing priorities drive people apart.

You know the saying: two heads are better than one. You might have another family member who's interested in losing weight, too. That's great news all around, but especially in the support department. If you're both motivated to slim down and

GET PSYCHED

"When I first took up jogging, my husband, an experienced runner, jogged along with me and encouraged me to enter short races. Once I got 'addicted' to the exercise, he no longer had to step in with support—how I felt after exercising was enough to motivate me to run." *—Jan B., Manchester, Connecticut*

ready to work together to achieve that goal, dieting becomes a less onerous task. The hard work of weight loss can be carried on two backs rather than one.

Family members can offer their support in quiet ways, which means it can be easily overlooked when you're expecting the big, grand gestures. For example, your spouse, who's not on a diet, who takes over the weekly grocery shopping, or the mother-in-law who makes sure there's always a low-cal dish on her table to accommodate your new eating plan.

Friends We usually don't get to pick who becomes a member of our family, except when we're choosing significant others and spouses (and inheriting their immediate families by association). Friendships, on the other hand, are handpicked. We might feel freer with our friends to show our true selves or express confidences than we do with parents or children. In other cases, friends support us when familial relationships are lacking or become damaged or fractured.

Behind many successful weight-loss endeavors stands a loyal friend. True friends are ready to cheer you on and motivate you, to pick you up when you're feeling down, to redirect you when you're lost, and they're proud when you reach your goals. Some friends don't mind if you call at 11 P.M. when you're having a chocolate craving; others will simply listen to your kvetching for hours on end until you feel better. Even if your friends aren't dieting, they'll often find ways to support you, such as offering to exercise with you at the gym or making sure you meet for lunch at a restaurant with a low-carb menu.

Bottom line: if you're not letting your friends know about your plans for weight loss, you're probably missing out on one of the best means of support.

Co-Workers They may not be your closest friends, but the people you work with every day can become assets to your weight-loss program. Because the health effects of obesity cost U.S. businesses $13 billion annually in health-care expenses and loss of productivity, many companies are implementing workplace weight-management programs for their employees. Although one recent study conducted by the American Association of Occupational Health Nurses showed that only 2 percent of the working population has participated in employer-sponsored plans, nearly 50 percent of those participants reached and maintained their weight-loss goals when they stuck with the program.

Workers take advantage of the support and camaraderie from co-workers who participate in the programs, as well as support from on-site professionals, such as nurses, dieticians, and fitness trainers. If you're not working for a Fortune 500 company with an on-site health club and a ready staff of health professionals, don't fret. Smaller companies can't compete with the array of support services a larger company can provide, but they can hold weight-loss challenges, provide fitness incentives, or negotiate a discount for employees with a local fitness center. Talk to your human resources personnel or a company director. And if that doesn't get you anywhere, start talking to your co-workers about setting up a weight-loss incentive program on your own.

Asking for Support

Asking for support can be tough for a lot of dieters. It means admitting to yourself and others that you've got a problem with your weight and you can't solve it on your own. It means being vulnerable, and allowing another person to examine your beliefs and behaviors about food. It means surrendering your pride, which can be a terrifying prospect for anyone, especially for a dieter who has eating issues built around shame, guilt, or other negative emotions.

Before you ask for support, you have to know what you want. Sit down and write out all the things that will help you meet your goals. Then figure out who best can help you with each item. What skills does each person in your life have? Is your girlfriend an enthusiastic cook who loves the challenge of discovering new recipes? Has your co-worker lost significant weight on the diet you're following?

The best way to ask for support is directly. If you've enlisted a close friend or relative, sit down with them and explain why you're dieting, what your goals are, and what you need from them to succeed. They'll probably be happy to help, although they may have some tough questions for you, such as, "Haven't you dieted before? What makes this time different?" Think about the questions they may ask beforehand so you're not put on the defensive. If you can't answer their questions, you can always tell them you'll get back with answers after you've thought about them.

The most important part of this conversation is being clear about what you want from them. "I want your support" is vague; "I need you to stop buying junk food for me because it's not part of my diet—here's what I'd like instead" is specific and action-oriented. "I want you to tell me when I'm eating something bad" is an open invitation for diet policing; it also puts too much responsibility on the other person for your behavior. A more effective request for support might be, "When I'm stressed about work, I tend to reach for cookies. Would you be open to letting me talk about work for a few minutes when I get home? I think that would help."

With an acquaintance or co-worker, asking for support doesn't have to be an event. "Hey, I'm having trouble finding the nutritional information for the food in the cafeteria—can you help?" will suffice. Who knows? From a simple question, a beautiful friendship may evolve.

Dealing With Sabotage

It can come in the form of a comment from your spouse that you look fine the way you are, so why do you need to spend an hour on your treadmill every day? It can be an irritation, such as your family monitoring everything that shows up on your plate at dinnertime. And it can hurt, such as with a best friend who criticizes the diet you're following and informs you over lunch why your diet's unscientific, unproven, and unhealthy. On top of that, she delivers her unsolicited opinion while scarfing down a rich chocolate dessert in front of you.

The good news about sabotaging behavior is that it's usually done unintentionally and without malice. The bad news is that even the most innocent comments or actions from others can send you into a tailspin if you aren't prepared for them. You're following new eating habits, which you've penned in your food journal and committed to memory. However, even people close to you may not be aware of your dietary changes, thus explaining why your spouse brings home a dozen warm, glazed doughnuts on Sunday morning. That's what he's always done and you've always enjoyed them. He may be genuinely confused about why you're suddenly angry with him.

The key is to let the people closest to you know as many details about your diet as you feel comfortable sharing so they can adjust their old assumptions and habits. Let your spouse know you appreciate his Sunday morning run to the doughnut shop, but you'd prefer a healthier treat, such as a whole-grain bagel with nonfat cream cheese from a local bakery.

Throwing the diet police off your trail can be a little trickier. Again, this kind of monitoring behavior is usually generated over concern for the dieter as a need to show support. This un-witting saboteur probably wants nothing more than to see you succeed with your weight-loss plans and thinks that by pointing out your stumbles and roadblocks, she's being "helpful." The key here is to sit down with the person and let her know exactly what you find helpful. If her policing makes you feel guilty about every morsel of food you put in your mouth or shames you into eating when you're alone, let her know how her behavior makes you feel. She's probably not purposely encouraging feelings of guilt and shame, and together you can come up with some ideas about how support can best be demonstrated. For example, you can agree to accept her monitoring only when you ask for it. Show your appreciation when she cooperates with your wishes; it will only encourage her to continue the supportive behavior you find most helpful.

GET PSYCHED

On sabotage: "I don't believe in it. It's all up to me in my book." —*Barb F., Louisville, Kentucky, 20 pounds lighter*

Trickiest of all is dealing with the saboteur who may be feeling ambivalent, even threatened, by your new eating habits and behaviors. If you and your best friend have always melted your sorrows away over hot fudge sundaes and now you're choosing diet sodas over ice cream, your friend could be dealing with emotions that have little to do with you and more with her own psychological issues. Seeing you take control of your eating could be reminding her of the lack of control in her own life. Or she may be wondering how secure your friendship is: what will change next between you two? Will you find new friends to replace her?

Sabotaging comments and behaviors should be approached and confronted with compassion, not anger. Let this person know how much you value your relationship, and explain how her behavior—the thinly veiled criticisms, her constant put-downs of your diet—hurts you and your friendship. You could point out the ways your relationship will improve through your weight loss. The time you've spent bonding over fatty, unhealthy foods could now be spent taking a healthful cooking class together through a local community center, for example.

The wiliest saboteur, of course, is your own mind, especially when you allow your thoughts and emotions to be controlled by another person's behavior or words. It's easy and convenient to blame someone else when you give in to temptation or go off your eating plan completely. Telling yourself, *It's his fault ... he shouldn't have brought those doughnuts into the house* or *Maybe I am too rigid about not eating desserts when I'm out with my friends* is easier than sitting down with someone to explain your needs or coming up with a plan to deal with negative comments ahead of time.

Also, keep in mind that no one is as interested in your diet as you are. It's easy to get caught up in a behavior that your friends, family, and acquaintances find irritating, such as announcing how many carbs every food item has before you let it pass your lips or other incessant chatter about diet and exercise. "Dieting is such an emotionally loaded issue," says Toni K. of New York City, who has lost 62 pounds through Weight Watchers, "that it's easy to forget not everyone is in the same place you are." What you may assume is sabotage behavior—for example, a friend who always changes the subject when you talk about your diet—is in fact his way of coping with behavior he finds irritating in you. The best way to find out what's going on is to ask. Ask "Is my food talk driving you nuts?" An explanation from you, "I'm sorry, but dieting is tough for me, and I forget not everyone is counting carbs," can be enough to ease the tension and get the relationship back on track.

Sabotage, whether real or imagined, intentional or hostile, is one of the things you'll find buried in the emotional minefield around your diet. You can either let yourself be blown away by the internal firestorm it generates or choose to deal with it by preparing for it ahead of time. It all comes down to personal responsibility. If you decide to eat those doughnuts, you have to accept that you made that decision, not your spouse. He may have carried them through the front door, but he certainly didn't force them down your throat.

Will a Support Group Help?

Research shows that support groups can play a positive role in helping dieters. Much of the work done by psychologist Michael Perri at the University of Florida shows that group support of long-term weight management is more effective than one-on-one support, even when subjects indicate a preference for one-on-one support. If you're a gregarious, social type of person by nature—an extrovert—there's a good chance you'll enjoy many aspects of the group meeting dynamic. You'll probably feel confident asking questions of the group's leader and comfortable approaching your peers for advice, support, and camaraderie. If you're the type who responds to accountability—knowing that other people are depending on you for support—you'll be apt to show up at meetings. And if you're hungry for support you're not finding at home or with friends, a support group will put you in contact with dozens, maybe even thousands, of other dieters who know how you're feeling.

Research shows that even quiet, solitary types—introverts—can find support in a live group setting. You're usually not required to speak; you can sit back and listen to the group leader share his experiences and take in the stories and tips others have to share. And it can be energizing to get out of the house, to feel as though you're part of a venture in which others are committed. And with the Internet providing so many avenues for support, quiet types can turn to their keyboards for help.

Another benefit of support groups is there's an opportunity to "give back" after you've achieved your weight-loss goal and kept if off. Peer and group leaders are often former dieters who've gotten results from the program, and they're eager to share what they've learned with the group. If you're satisfied with the results you're getting with the group, you can strive to become a group leader yourself.

But groups do have their drawbacks. Live group meetings can cost you money, and commercial diet-support groups often push their own products at meetings, which can drive your costs up even farther. They can become slavish, even cultist, in their dedication to a diet's principles or with a charismatic group leader. Deviation from the party line can earn you a blank stare, ridicule, flaming (if you're online), or other uncomfortable reactions.

For example, Toni K. of New York City became disillusioned with her Weight Watchers group leader when Toni mentioned a *Wall Street Journal* article that reported there was no scientific proof that drinking lots of water helped dieters lose weight. "Weight Watchers tells you to drink six eight-ounce glasses a day," she says, "so the group leader got defensive. She went off on a tirade about journalists."

I'm nervous I'll have to tell everyone at a group meeting how much I really weigh. What can I expect?

"At a Weight Watchers meeting, you'll find a very supportive and nurturing environment for new and returning members," says Amy B. Crane of Erie, Pennsylvania, a Weight Watchers lifetime member since 2003. "There is never any pressure to speak or to reveal what you weigh. The leader generally has a topic, which could be anything from dealing with too much food over the holidays, exercising, or choosing healthier food at restaurants. They'll talk some about that topic, ask questions or ask for feedback from anyone who wants to volunteer an answer. Usually plenty of people want to talk; listening to them is a great way to pick up tips that really work in people's lives. And when you reach a milestone, such as losing 5 or 10 pounds or more, you'll be recognized and given a sticker. People will applaud you, which is really encouraging."

Another dieter, Deb E. of Sydney, Australia, joined Weight Watchers with the goal of losing a few pounds around her belly. When she stood on the scale at the first meeting, the group leader told her she was within the healthy weight range for her height.

GET PSYCHED

"It takes a strong person to take what they need from a formal group meeting and discard the rest."
—*Toni K., New York City, 62 pounds lighter*

"Then she proceeded to tell me I only needed to lose five kilos," says Deb. "It was the 'need' that miffed me. I mean, I may want to lose some weight, but clearly by their measures I don't 'need' to. Plus, if I got down to the weight target she set for me, I would have been at the very bottom of the healthy range and under the weight where you are even eligible to join Weight Watchers."

You might not care for or connect with the group's members or leader, which can cause you to believe group support is not for you. You can get around this by sticking with the group for a couple meetings and then checking how you feel; perhaps that first meeting you attended wasn't an accurate representation of the usual dynamic. If you don't warm up after a few meetings, check out other meetings around town. Sometimes it's a matter of finding the right fit. After Toni K.'s chilly encounter with her group leader, she began attending meetings conducted by another group leader who was more accepting of different views.

Local Groups Obesity is at epidemic levels in the United States, and chances are your community has at least one— probably several—weight-loss group meetings to offer. Check bulletin boards at your public library or supermarket, the community calendar listing in your local newspaper, or ask friends and neighbors for their recommendations.

Popular weight-loss groups include Weight Watchers, Overeaters Anonymous, TOPS Club, Inc., and hospital-based programs.

Weight Watchers (www.weightwatchers.com). The grandmother of all weight-loss programs, Weight Watchers meetings can be found from Calais, Maine, to Fairbanks, Alaska, and beyond. One caveat: meetings focus on dieters who are following Weight Watchers–endorsed diet plans.

Overeaters Anonymous (www.oa.org). Based on the precepts of Alcoholics Anonymous, Overeaters Anonymous supports those who struggle with compulsive overeating, including binge and emotional eating. The website includes a meeting locator tool and a list of Internet-based meetings held in real time.

There are no dues or fees, although contributions are accepted at meetings.

TOPS Club, Inc. (www.tops.org). TOPS (Taking Off Pounds Sensibly) is a fee-based nonprofit group dedicated to supporting people of all ages, sizes, and shapes from all walks of life to lose weight. More than 200,000 members in 10,000 chapters in the United States, Canada, and abroad attend weekly meetings that include private weigh-ins.

Hospital-based programs. Check out newsletters and bulletin boards at your local hospital, or ask your physician for a recommendation.

Internet Groups If your schedule doesn't permit a weekly weight-loss support meeting or you prefer anonymity, the Internet can put you in contact with thousands of other dieters around the world, all from the comfort of your home or office 24/7. Some groups, bulletin boards, and listservs are administered by for-profit weight-loss organizations, but many others are put together by like-minded dieters or nonprofits. When you start searching the Internet, you'll soon discover there's a support group for every kind of dieter and every type of diet.

Here are some starting points for your Internet research:

- Usenet/news groups. Search groups.google.com. Relevant groups include alt.support.diet, alt.support.diet. weightwatchers, alt.support.obesity, and alt.recovery. compulsive-eat.

- groups.yahoo.com. There are more than 2,000 groups listed under the weight-loss category, and another 800+ groups for specific diets. You'll also find groups for obesity, eating disorders, and other weight issues.

- www.diettalk.com/forums. An online peer support group with dozens of subforums: a low-carb group; an emergency support group; groups for people dealing with body-image, motivation, and weight-maintenance issues; and groups for teens, seniors, and dieters who have 100+ pounds to lose.

- weightloss.about.com/mpboards.htm. This weight-loss forum is a component of About.com's weight-loss topic. You'll need to register to post to this active forum, where members share victories, before and after photos, and recipe tips.

- Commercial sites. Websites such as Diet.com, eDiets.com, Atkins.com, and DrSears.com (the Zone Diet) have very active forums, as well as some great web-based tools such as diet journals, body fat calculators, and meal plans. Some boards, such as the one on eDiets, have a subscription cost; others, such as the one on Dr. Sears's site, are free. The catch? With the diet-specific boards, including the Atkins one and The Zone, you're subject to prevailing group wisdom and advertising, which can be irritating if you happen to disagree with it.

- Diet-specific sites. Plug the name of your diet into Google, and you'll find dozens of support forums. They're usually free, but you probably have to register if you want to post on them.

> **WEB TALK:** The Tufts University Nutrition Navigator rates and scores more than 200 weight-loss websites and provides brief reviews and recommendations:
>
> ➤ www.navigator.tufts.edu

Diet/Exercise Buddies A diet or exercise buddy is an excellent source of support when you're dieting. Someone who is as motivated as you are to eat well, exercise right, and really change his or her life can help you achieve goals you've not been able to meet in the past.

you're not alone

When Jamie U. was looking for support to stay on her diet, she only had to walk down the street to find it.

Late in 2004, this stay-at-home mother from Austin, Texas, rounded up 10 of her neighbors for a diet and exercise buddy group to support each other as they pursued individual weight-loss and fitness goals. She was inspired by the television show *Dr. Phil*, which urges dieters to form buddy groups for support. "Getting together as a group has forced us to face what we're eating, how we're exercising, and it also keeps us motivated," she says.

At the first meeting, the group—all women between the ages of 27 and 35—set general guidelines and expectations. "Some of us want to weigh in," Jamie says, "while others don't. There's no pressure to follow a certain kind of diet; some of us are just trying to exercise more and eat better." The meetings rotate between members' homes, and one person brings a low-cal snack along with its recipe. Food and/or fitness journals are de rigueur, and at the meeting they're discussed and reviewed by the group. During the week, members are always in touch by e-mail. Jamie says, "Some of us work outside the home, so it's easier to plan things that way, or just give each other encouragement." One Saturday morning, the group got together to have their body fat and physical measurements taken by one member's friend, who happened to be a health professional.

Jamie adds, "We were friends before we started the group, so that has made our commitment to the group stronger. These are people who are making you get real about weight loss, who see your body every day, and for sure, it makes a big difference."

Enlisting the aid of a diet or exercise buddy doesn't have to be a formal affair, although that's certainly one way to do it. Look around your neighborhood: is there a neighbor who walks up and down the street at the same time every day? Ask if he'd mind if you joined him. You can strike up conversations with people you see every day at the gym. Even knowing there's a friendly person working out on the elliptical trainer next to yours can be enough to get you out of bed in the morning.

If you're looking for a more formal arrangement, check out these resources:

- Diettalk.com's Diet Buddy Forum (www.diettalk.com/ forums/forumdisplay.php?f=24) is loaded with posts from people around the country looking for virtual and real-time diet buddies.
- MyDietBuddy.com is another Internet-based site that matches up dieters for virtual support. There's no charge for the support, but membership requires filling out a survey.
- The Diet Buddies (www.thedietbuddies.bravepages. com/home.htm) is another web-based matching service. Started by two friends (and diet buddies), this site is free and includes a chat room and newsletter.
- Food and Diet (www.foodanddiet.com/NewFiles/ exercisebuddies-available.html) offers an exercise and diet buddy matching service, searchable by state.

What You Can Do

Fortunately, support resources are rich and varied for dieters. With a little effort and maybe a dash of courage, you'll probably find what you need close to your home or office. Barring that, effective, meaningful support can come from relative strangers— even through your computer.

☐ Reach out to everyone you know for support. Losing weight isn't something to be ashamed about. Overweight is a condition affecting millions of Americans, so chances are good someone you know can understand and support your weight-loss program.

☐ Find a local diet-support group that meets your specific needs, and attend a few meetings to see if it's a good fit.

☐ If your schedule is already packed with commitments, investigate Internet-based means of support.

☐ Know what kind of support you need to meet the goals of your diet. Write down a wish list of actions and behaviors you'd find most helpful from your family, friends, and other people you meet on your weight-loss journey. Now figure out how you can get those needs met.

☐ Work out ahead of time how you'll handle people who aren't supporting you the way you'd like to be supported. You'll be able to act rationally rather than react emotionally.

☐ When you're comfortable receiving support, consider reaching out to support others with their weight-loss efforts. You can volunteer to become a peer leader at your group meeting, or simply stand up and share your experience with new dieters.

☐ If you're not finding the support you need at home, among your friends, or within your community, start your own support group, inviting anyone you think would benefit.

☐ Remember, no one is as invested in your diet plan as you are. Slip-ups and bad decisions are your responsibility. Likewise, the victories and goals met come down to you and your consistent efforts.

Helping Someone You Love Lose Weight

n my extended family is a relative I'll call Betty. Betty has been in good shape for most of her life. In her 70s, she still wore shorts and took pride in her slim, toned "dancer legs." She has never had to worry about her weight: "I just eat what I want and never seem to gain."

Her three children, however, have grappled with weight problems most of their lives. When her children were young, she enrolled them in dance classes and organized sports, hoping those activities would encourage weight loss. Today, when she has guests, Betty points to a framed photo of her youthful daughter. "Even then she was fat," Betty says. "She must have gotten it from her father."

When one of her sons visits from out of town, Betty gives him a hug and steps back. Then her gaze drops to his midsection, and she says, "Boy, you've packed on more weight." She usually delivers the comment with a playful poke at his belly. Later, when another family member points out that her comments were embarrassing and hurtful to her son, she shrugs them off. "I'm his mother," she says. "I can say things like that. And besides, he *is* fat."

Betty doesn't limit her critiques to her own children, however. Her teenage grandson is overweight. Betty started needling him about why he wasn't thin like his cousins. His parents pleaded with Betty to stop the comparisons, but Betty insisted she was "just trying to help."

Betty doesn't understand why her grandson has cut off contact with her. She doesn't understand why her own children don't visit as much as she'd like. When I finally pointed out that her comments about their weight probably had something to do with the emotional distance, she looked baffled. "But they *are* overweight. I'm not saying anything that's not true."

Support or Sabotage?

When you live with someone who needs to lose weight or you have a friend whose health is compromised by obesity, of course you want to do everything you can to help. You care about people you love, and it's natural to want to do or say something that will make a difference in their lives. Or you may be someone who cares about how everyone eats. Maybe health and wellness are so important to you that you feel it's your mission to educate everyone about diet and exercise. You figure you're doing the stranger in the grocery store a service when you point out how many trans fats are in the cookies she's buying.

But weight is a sensitive issue. Some of the worst insults thrown around involve weight or size: *fatso, porker, pig, whale, blimp, big fat slob*, and a host of other derisive names. Anyone who has spent a lifetime overweight or obese has probably had most of these awful epithets hurled at them. Even *fat* is derogatory.

Chances are that any discussion of size or weight is going to be a loaded subject. It may seem as though your comment about your brother's growing girth doesn't bother him, but it probably does, even if he doesn't show it. Unlike many other health conditions, overweight and obesity isn't something he can shield from the world. He knows he has a weight problem, and so does everyone else who sees him. Pointing out what's blatantly obvious serves no purpose.

Often a dieter's loved ones are unwitting saboteurs because they frequently transform themselves into "diet cops." Their intentions are usually good, but their questions, such as "Are those french fries on your diet?" or comments such as, "You skipped your walk yesterday and the day before. I hope you're not quitting this diet already," are not usually what the dieter wants—or really needs—to hear.

> ## GET PSYCHED
>
> "The less you judge other people by the way they look, the less judged by others you will feel yourself."
> —*Victoria Moran in* Fit from Within

Sometimes a dieter will ask you to "help" them. You interpret that request as an invitation to step in when you see them doing something "wrong" or "bad." When you get this kind of request, ask the dieter to be very specific about what they consider helpful. "Help" means different things to different people. You may think you're being helpful by reprimanding them for skipping a workout, but they may interpret that "help" as annoying.

Diet policing usually backfires and produces the opposite effect the diet cop intended. For example, a wife criticizes her husband for eating cheese and crackers in front of the TV. "You're not going to lose weight eating *those*," she says. He wearily returns the cheese to the refrigerator and the crackers to the cupboard. The wife is shocked when but a few days later, she catches him eating the cheese and crackers in his home workshop.

Whether you're a friend or a family member of a dieter—or even a stranger—resist the urge to police. You can use other, more effective ways to offer your support to someone you love and care about or show your enthusiasm about health and diet.

Another way family members and friends try to show support is by leaving out articles about the benefits of weight loss. Or they'll e-mail a news story to a dieter about the dangers of the diet they're following. You may think this subtle approach is a perfectly reasonable way to get someone to take action or show you care about their health, but it usually only succeeds in breeding resentment.

you're not alone

When her mother's friend asked her to join Weight Watchers in January 2004, Liz L., 24, was a bit taken aback. "It was like, *Hmmm, someone's noticing I need to lose weight.*" Rather than take offense, the Boise, Idaho woman decided to think about it for a night. She said, "I knew my mother's friend had my best interests at heart and that she wanted someone to do the program with her." She decided to sign up and told herself she'd give it a week to see how it worked out.

Liz admits she was daunted at the first meeting. She was one of the youngest members there and felt out of place. "The group leader explained the program and I thought, *I can't do this, I can't watch everything that goes past my lips for the next 50 years.*" She enjoyed going out with her friends at night and on the weekends, and the thought of giving all that up for a lifetime of calorie counting scared her. But Liz stuck to the plan for a week. She was pleasantly shocked when she stood

Every dieter has challenges. Your best friend's challenge may be getting to the gym on a regular basis. It probably doesn't help her if you boast, "Oh, going to the gym is never a hassle for me. I just love it. Look at my arms. See the definition in my biceps." What may be "easy" for you to achieve may be a monumental difficulty for her—and vice versa. You have to understand that losing weight is different for everyone and treat your friends, family, and spouses with empathy and kindness.

Communicating Concern

In a poll of 1,000 women conducted by *People* magazine in 2000, 37 percent said their spouses would like them to lose weight. In a 2001 poll of 1,000 husbands and wives conducted by *Reader's Digest,* a quarter of both sexes responded that they can't discuss their spouse's need to lose weight with them. (In

on the scale at the next meeting and saw that she'd lost 5 pounds. "I thought, *Wow, this is great!"*

Over the next year, Liz continued with the Weight Watchers program and lost 20 more pounds. As the weight dropped away, she started telling her friends about her diet, and she appreciated the small ways they supported her. "They would let me drive when we went out," she says, "so I could steer the car to the restaurant that was better for my diet, or leave early." Eventually, some of her co-workers joined the program, and now they walk together at lunchtime.

How has the loss of 25 pounds impacted her life? There's a long list: "I've been working out," says Liz. "I can get through a spinning class, which I couldn't have done a year ago. I don't get tired, and I have more energy. I'm much happier. People notice. It's really nice to go to a family function and have them say, 'Wow, you look really good!'"

fact, losing weight came up as one of the top nagging topics in marriages.) In another interesting survey done by the British women's magazine *She*, 55 percent of women said they'd rather be lied to about their weight than told the truth.

So with all this worry about saying or doing the wrong thing, what's the best way to communicate your concern to someone who needs to lose weight? Take your focus off them, and put it on yourself.

I'm really worried about my wife, who just turned 50. It seems like she put on 50 or 60 pounds in the last couple years. I notice she can't walk up stairs without gasping for breath. I keep telling her she needs to see a doctor, but she gets angry with me. What else can I do besides nag?

"Gasping for breath can sometimes be as simple as being de-conditioned and overweight, but it can also be a sign of other serious medical conditions. Tell your wife in a loving, nonconfrontational manner—this is key—that you are concerned about what you're noticing and invite her to see her doctor for a checkup. Ideally, it would be nice for you to have some time with your wife and her doctor to discuss these issues as a starting point. The patient/doctor relationship is pretty sacrosanct, but sometimes a meeting can be arranged for the end of a session, as long as the patient and the doctor are both aware of this beforehand. More time needs to be set aside for this visit, which is why the doctor should know this up front. If an end-of-session meeting isn't possible, sometimes a follow-up appointment can be arranged.

"Remember that 'turnabout is fair play.' Sometimes such a meeting can be viewed as less threatening if both spouses agree to checkups and the other spouse is given the same opportunity to meet with the doctor afterward. An agreement like this can help everyone feel empowered and on equal footing about the discussion of medical issues. While I wouldn't recommend this type of discussion at most visits, the occasional partner/partner/doctor visit can allay fears and lead to better communication." *—Mark B. Davidson, M.D., a Westford, Massachusetts–based physician associated with Emerson Hospital, Concord, Massachusetts*

Offer opportunities for things you can do together rather than make suggestions about changes he or she can make on their own. If you notice your spouse is putting on weight, you could try something such as, "I'm going to start walking after dinner. Want to join me?" or "I noticed that the community center is offering a couples, low-fat, Mexican cooking class. Because we both love Mexican food, why don't we sign up?" If you and a friend always meet for fast food, suggest you start meeting at another restaurant that offers healthier food choices you can both enjoy.

Verbal Strategies It may be obvious to you that someone needs to lose weight, but if they're not ready, chances are that your begging, pleading, and nagging will contribute little to their making changes. People tend not to make major life changes because of nagging. Research conducted by the National Weight Control Registry (NWCR) in Denver shows that men tend to make changes because of a specific health problem—they're having trouble with their knees, for example, so they begin to lose weight to make them feel better. Women, on the other hand, tend to have more feelings attached to weight loss—they're feeling wiped out or feeling like they don't want to carry extra weight around.

However, there are still ways you can verbally "help" or motivate someone to get to that place:

- When talking about diets or overweight, avoid using the words *should* or *could*, which can sometimes sound accusatory.

- When someone brings up their weight concerns with you, resist the temptation to jump in with your advice. Listen, instead, and if you have to talk, ask questions. If they're telling you they're ready to lose weight, ask them what they need you to do to help.

307

- Remember that being someone's mother, father, sister, lover, spouse, or best friend does not give you the right to deliver your opinion when it hasn't been asked for.

- Instead of asking the person why they haven't worked out all week, say, "I'm going for my walk, and I'd love the company. Would you join me?"

- Take the focus off weight when complimenting a friend or family member. Try "Wow, you look terrific!" versus "You've lost weight!" and see how the dieter responds. Chances are, he or she will positively glow with the compliment and be eager to share with you his or her weight-loss progress.

GET PSYCHED

"One day a neighbor mentioned to me, 'You know, every morning I see you out there, and you look like you're really enjoying your jog. That's nice to see.' It made me feel good inside because in the beginning, jogging wasn't fun for me. I realized then how far I'd come." –Jan, Manchester, Connecticut

Nonverbal Strategies Here are some nonverbal ways to support someone you care about who needs to lose weight or who is dieting:

Show your concern by example. Take care of your own body with diet and exercise. Many times dieters are resentful of family members and friends because they engage in the very same behaviors they're lecturing the dieter to avoid.

If you're the one who does the cooking in your home, look for ways to incorporate the dieter's needs into your meals.

Look at the habits you've adopted with your friends and family, and see if they need to be changed for new circumstances. If you've always bought chocolates for your wife on her birthday, she may find this year's gift of Godiva a sabotaging move.

Coping with Emotions and Mood Swings

Losing weight is one of the toughest tasks we can accomplish. Sometimes dieting leaves us feeling not so great, physically or mentally. When we first start a weight-loss plan, our stomachs aren't used to smaller portions, so we feel hungry much of the time—ravenously so. We can get cranky when we're trying to cut back on substances such as sugars and caffeine or regulate the intake of certain nutrients such as carbohydrates and fats. Some of us are sensitive to the toxins we're eliminating from our bodies when we burn off fat, so we feel weak, tired, spacey, or headachy as a result.

On top of this, we're battling our bodies' cravings for the foods we're trying not to eat or drink: potato chips, ice cream, chocolate, soft drinks, and fast-food hamburgers. It's a physical challenge as well as a mental one. All day we're around people who aren't dieting—people who are eating the foods we have given up. We bring our soup, salad, and diet soda to work and sit there drooling at our co-workers' supersize burgers and fries.

> **GET PSYCHED**
>
> "Sensitivity is an admirable quality ... The problem comes in not knowing how to control its intensity or channel its course."
> —*Victoria Moran in* Fit from Within

After work, we head off to the gym, and while other people around us seem to enjoy the treadmills and weights, we're not at that point yet. Exercise is still hard. We feel like we're going through the motions, and we're not seeing any results. Inside, we know it takes time to get fit, but it doesn't make exercising any easier.

Then we come home. We step on the scale and do a double-take at the number. Only ½ pound lost since last week? We're dismayed. We're angry. We feel like giving up. That's when our

309

spouse cheerfully reminds us it's our turn to take out the garbage. And that's when we explode.

Living with a dieter can be challenging. Beyond the occasional moodiness, there are the frequent bouts of self-absorption, when all the dieter can talk about is his progress, his calorie intake, how much he's lost in the last 24 hours, and other less-than-scintillating details of his weight-loss plan. He even reverses the diet cop scenario and starts pointing out why *you* shouldn't be eating the food in front of you.

Living with a dieter can test your nerves, but it's survivable:

- Try not to take their moods personally, and remember that developing new eating habits tends to get easier as time passes.
- Let dieters who police your choices know that although you appreciate their interest in food and diet, you'll let them know how you want to be helped when you're changing your diet.
- Remind the dieter you have challenges, too: But I'm stressed about this project I'm working on, and I want to decompress when I get home. Can we talk about your diet after the kids have gone to bed?"

Children and Teens

As the number of overweight and obese children and teens in the United States continues to grow, parents find themselves not only monitoring their own dietary intakes, but the diets of their offspring as well. According to the Center for National Health Statistics, the percentage of school-age children ages 6 to 11 who are overweight more than doubled between the late 1970s and 2000, rising from 6.5 percent to 15.3 percent. The percentage of overweight adolescents ages 12 to 19 tripled from 5 percent to 15.5 percent during the same time period. Today, the American Obesity Association estimates approximately 30.3 percent of children ages 6 to 11 are overweight, and 15.3 percent are obese. For adolescents (ages 12 to 19), 30.4 percent are overweight and 15.5 percent are obese. Doctors who were seeing only adults for obesity-related type 2 diabetes and hypertension are now treating increasing numbers of children and adolescents for these conditions.

Unfortunately, many parents pass on a tendency for overweight and obesity to their children, either through genetics, environment, or a combination of both. A research study led by Robert Berkowitz, M.D., at the Children's Hospital of Philadelphia showed that by age 6, children of overweight mothers were 15 times more likely to be obese than children of lean mothers. The study followed 70 children over 6 years at the hospital. Thirty-three children had overweight moms and 37 had lean ones. During the first 2 years, there was little difference between the weight and body composition of the two groups. But the children who had overweight moms had greater overall weight by age 4 and both greater weight and body fat by age 6. "There appears to be an interaction between the genes that control body weight and environmental factors such as increased intake of sweets and fats, as well as inactivity, all of which are associated with the development of childhood obesity," noted Albert J. Stunkard, M.D., of the University of Pennsylvania School of Medicine, a co-author of the study. The researchers concluded that prevention efforts should begin by age 4 for overweight children of overweight moms.

Dr. Osama Hamdy, director of the Obesity Clinic, assistant investigator in the Section on Clinical Research at Joslin Diabetes Center and an instructor in medicine at Harvard Medical School in Boston, Massachusetts, is passionate about the responsibility adults should take in their children's diets. "We are heading toward a crisis," he says. "Look at a kids' menu at a restaurant. What are the options? It's a burger, a hot dog, chicken nuggets, or pizza. There's rarely a salad or other healthy choices. We are forcing kids to eat the wrong foods, and that's why children and adolescents are becoming overweight or obese." Hamdy is not only passionate about this subject as a researcher, but also as a father of young children.

When you're watching your weight as an adult, you have more resources at your disposal: you can create strategies to help you cope with psychological weaknesses and temptations. Kids tend not to have those skills. Young children haven't developed the maturity to ignore the advertising bombardments for sweet or fatty junk foods, or the wisdom that informs them a turkey sandwich will ultimately give them more nutrition than a supersize fast-food meal. Moreover, you can't always be there 24/7 to help your child make the best food choices. You're often at the mercy of your school system's lunch program or the judgment of other parents. The best you feel you can do is teach them good eating habits at home, and even that can be hard. Indeed, your sphere of influence over your child's eating habits diminishes with every passing year.

GET PSYCHED

"I want my children to have a positive association with healthy foods, so we do food associations at meals. I'll ask my son, 'What do you think pilots like to eat?' if we're having broccoli, and we'll decide that pilots eat broccoli because it's good for their brains."
—Meredith, New Jersey

In 2004, Kelly Brownell, Ph.D., director of the Yale Center for Eating and Weight Disorders, wrote an informative and controversial book called *Food Fight*, in which he examines the food industry's role in America's obesity crisis. Although he points out that parents aren't immune from the same toxic health environments affecting their kids, he does note that some practices have been proven to help combat childhood overweight and obesity:

Breast-feeding. Studies show that children who are breast-fed tend to have lower rates of obesity. Moreover, breast-fed children tend to be more adventurous eaters. This may be attributed to the variabilities in the taste of a mother's milk supply because of what she eats. (Note to breast-feeding moms: eat your veggies!)

Reduced television/sedentary activities at home. Brownell recommends parents take televisions out of children's bedrooms, turn off televisions at mealtimes, and reduce the time spent with computers and computer games.

> **GET PSYCHED**
>
> "When my sons were young, I prepared cut-up raw vegetables, fruits, and healthy dips for them to snack on. Those foods were always available in our house. Now my sons are 18 and 20, and both are big vegetable eaters who are in excellent shape. I think making healthy foods available for children makes a tremendous difference in how they eat as adults."
> —*Jan, 48, Manchester, Connecticut*

Physical activity. When your child spends less time in front of the television or engaging in sedentary activities, she'll have more time to engage in activities that get her active and moving.

> **WEB TALK:** Check out the American Obesity Association's fact sheet on childhood obesity at:
> ▲ www.obesity.org/subs/childhood/

At Home As a parent, there are lots of things you can do rather than say to encourage children to achieve and maintain a healthy weight:

- Substitute activities for food when spending time together as a family. Rather than treat the whole family to ice cream on Friday evening, head to a local skating rink or go for a walk together in a park.

313

- If you're trying to lose weight with a healthful, balanced diet, there's no reason why your children can't eat the same food, too. Encourage them to eat whole grains, lean meats, fruits, and vegetables along with you.

- Plan an active vacation together. Learn to ski together as a family, or schedule in activities such as horseback riding lessons or berry picking at a you-pick farm. Do something fun, such as taking trapeze lessons!

- Let children help you prepare healthy meals for the whole family. Young children can pick cherry tomatoes in the garden; older children can help wash produce and tear up lettuce.

- Dine together. Turn off the television. Focus on eating slowly and enjoying each other's company.

- Practice portion control. Let children start out with a small serving; they can always have more if they're still hungry.

- Disband the clean-plate club. If your child says she's not hungry, don't force her to eat. All this does is teach her to ignore her body and brain's natural appetite and satiety signals, which will cause more problems as she ages. Instead, focus on controlling portions, tasting small amounts of new foods, and keeping mealtime stress-free.

- Avoid rewarding or punishing children with food. Again, this sets up children for emotional eating patterns later in life.

At School Today, many schoolchildren are subject to policies that discourage healthy eating and exercise and encourage overweight and obesity. In a poll conducted by the American Obesity Association, parents rated how well their children's school programs were teaching good patterns of eating and physical activity to prevent obesity. Thirty-five percent rated the schools' efforts as "poor," "nonexistent," or "don't know." Moreover, schools are free to bypass the U.S. Department of Agriculture's (USDA) dietary guidelines for foods sold à la carte, food sold in snack bars, and food sold through vending machines, which means children have more opportunities than ever to fill their growing bodies with cookies, chips, and soda rather than healthier foods.

> **WEB TALK:** Find tips on how to get involved with providing children healthy lunches at:
> www.fns.usda.gov/tn/Parents/lunch.html

Sadly, some parents fail to grasp the gravity of childhood nutrition and fitness on overweight and obesity. In a case that shows just how prickly some parents are about changing the status quo, a New Jersey mother of two young children approached school officials in her upscale suburban town about improving school lunches and discouraging rewards of snacks such as Starburst Fruit Chews and doughnut holes in the classrooms. Her suggestions were met with such disdain and even hostility among parents that the story made the local papers. The concerned mother was labeled "the cupcake cop." One newspaper quoted a parent who thought the mother should move back to Atlanta. A school official pointed out to reporters that the mother rented rather than owned her home in the town, suggesting she had no right to voice her concerns.

In June 2000, the American Academy of Family Physicians, the American Academy of Pediatrics, the American Dietetic Association, the National Hispanic Medical Association, the National Medical Association, and the USDA proposed a "Prescription for Change: Ten Keys to Promote Healthy Eating in Schools" to be used for guidance in school nutrition programs. Their prescription ...

- Students, parents, food service staff, educators, and community leaders will be involved in assessing the schools' eating environment and developing a shared vision and an action plan to achieve it.
- Adequate funds will be provided by local, state, and federal sources to ensure that the total school environment supports the development of healthy eating patterns.
- Behavior-focused nutrition education will be integrated into the curriculum from pre-K through grade 12. Staff who provide nutrition education will have appropriate training.
- School meals will meet the USDA nutrition standards as well as provide sufficient choices, including new foods and foods prepared in new ways, to meet the taste preferences of diverse student populations.
- All students will have designated lunch periods of sufficient length to enjoy eating healthful foods with friends. These lunch periods will be scheduled as near the middle of the school day as possible.
- Schools will provide enough serving areas to ensure student access to school meals with a minimum of wait time.
- There will be adequate space to accommodate all students as well as pleasant surroundings that reflect the value of the social aspects of eating.
- Students, teachers, and community volunteers who practice healthy eating will be encouraged to serve as role models in the school dining areas.
- If foods are sold in addition to National School Lunch Program meals, they will be from the Food Guide Pyramid's five major food groups. This practice will foster healthy eating patterns.

- Decisions regarding the sale of foods in addition to the National School Lunch Program meals will be based on nutrition goals, not on profit making.

If you're concerned about the quality of food and physical education at your child's school, speak up. Ask questions. Talk to other parents about their concerns, and join together to work on behalf of the children's best interests. It may not be easy, and you could be met with hostility, but overweight and obesity are public health problems that affect your children. The attitudes and habits your children pick up now are the ones they'll carry with them into adulthood.

What You Can Do

There's not a lot you can do to make a spouse, relative, or friend decide to lose weight. There's also not much you can do to "make" someone stick to a diet. The best you can do is respect their choices and hope that by taking care of your own health, you'll set an example of wellness that will motivate them to reconsider their health.

☐ Practice compassion. Accept that other people may not be at a place in their lives where they're ready to take control of their weight.

☐ Offer your dieting advice and success story only when you're asked specifically about it. Let them know that you have every confidence that they, too, can have the same success you've had.

☐ Share your success story to motivate others to create their own successes. Tell them what you did, what your challenges were, and how you feel now that you've lost the weight.

☐ Try not to dismiss the challenges other dieters have. They may have a challenge with something you felt was easy to overcome, but that doesn't mean it's any less of a challenge for them.

☐ Download a list of questions to assess your child's school lunch program from www.healthinschools.org/parents/lunch.htm.

☐ When you want to offer help, choose actions over words. If you would like your spouse to exercise more, ask if he wants to walk with you. If your girlfriend is tired of dieting, offer to listen to her complaints and resist the urge to jump in with solutions.

Adjusting to Permanent Weight Loss

You did it! After months, maybe even years of slow, steady progress, you've reached your goal weight. You've worked hard. You've persevered when you felt like quitting. When you fell down, you got back up. You've developed new, healthy habits to replace old behaviors that contributed to your weight gain.

This is where most diet books cut you loose and send you off into the sunset. You're considered "cured." You're one of the lucky few, a maintainer. Now all that's left for you to do is go out there and conquer the world.

Were it that easy. You may have changed your size and shape radically. You may have changed a lot of your behaviors and many of your attitudes about food, exercise, dieting, health, and more. But not everything about you has changed. In many ways, you're essentially the person you were before you lost weight. When you realize this, it can bring up a lot of scary feelings: anxiety, fear, anger, disappointment. On top of this, you may still be thinking of yourself as an overweight person, which trips you up now that you're at a healthier weight. Things "normal people" take for granted are confusing to you—everything from shopping for clothes and accepting compliments to even sitting down or standing up.

You're supposedly at the end of the journey, but really, you're just at the beginning. And unlike the last few months or past years, you no longer have a clear roadmap. How will you maintain your weight? Now that you don't have goals and milestones to work for, how will you motivate yourself to keep up the good work? Questions and worries such as these can be scary.

Let's talk about the challenges of finally mastering weight loss and how you can enjoy what you've worked so hard for and dreamed about for so long to achieve.

Reshaping Your Thoughts

You believed when you finally lost the weight, your life would change dramatically. You may have lived for years with this belief, dreaming of the day when you'd be thin and what your new life would finally be like.

Losing weight *will* improve your life. You'll certainly be healthier and reduce your chances of developing serious, life-threatening diseases. And you may very well be happier. You certainly won't have many of the problems and challenges you struggled with when you were heavier.

But like lottery winners, successful dieters often discover life doesn't change that much with the stroke of good fortune—or in this case, with the stigma of overweight removed. Being slim and healthy doesn't mean everyone will automatically like you. You will discover that people can still be rude and unkind. If you were in a bad relationship when you were heavy, chances are, it's going to be a bad relationship now that you're lighter, too. If you didn't get along with people at work when you were heavy, you will probably not get along with them afterward either.

This is why it's important to reshape your thinking after weight loss, about everything from how you feel about yourself inside to the way you relate with and interact with others—strangers as well as the people you love the most.

"Fat" Thinking

Do any of the following scenarios sound familiar?

- When you walk into a crowded restaurant, you automatically let your dining companions walk ahead of you. Why? Sometimes you forget the girth that used to push everyone out of the way is gone.

- For a second, you hesitate before sitting down on a folding chair, or worry what people will think if you go for seconds at a banquet. Then you realize that at your current weight, you probably won't break the chair or cause anyone to stare if you get more food.

- A group of construction workers showers you with wolf whistles on the way to work. The first thing you think is, *This must be a joke. They're just making fun of me.*

- You automatically reach for the styles of clothes you wore when you were heavier: loose-fitting tunic shirts, baggy gym clothes, and elastic-waist pants.

You're at your ideal weight on the outside, but on the inside, you're still thinking "fat." Letting go of that "fat" thinking takes

GET PSYCHED

"I still sometimes consider myself obese, but recently I had an epiphany. I went to buy some pants. When I went to the 'big and tall' section of the store, I couldn't find my size. I asked the salesperson to help me find a size 40/42. He said, 'Sir, you're in the wrong section. You'll have to go to the normal section for that size.' I made him take me to the other section. And there they were, pants in my size in all different colors and styles. I was just stunned and had to explain to him all I'd gone through to get to that section." *—Bo McCoy, Capistrano Beach, California*

time, and many people never completely eradicate it. If you've been overweight or obese for most of your life, fat thinking served a valuable purpose. It helped you cope with the world, and it became automatic.

But now that you've lost weight, "fat" thinking no longer supports who you are. It can cause you to stay in your shell or further reinforce your insecurities. You may become suspicious of someone who only has good intentions. What can you do to cope with "fat" thinking?

Catch those moments you find yourself falling into "fat" thinking, and write about them in your journal. What were the circumstances leading up to that thought? What assumptions did you make about the situation? What made you realize these assumptions were invalid? How do you feel now?

Observe how other people behave in the situations that bring out "fat" thinking, and mimic their behaviors. What happens when you smile and say "thank you" after a compliment?

You may automatically think someone is being rude to you at a store because you're overweight. Most of the time people are rude because of something that has nothing to do with you.

Your "fat" thinking can help you become even more aware of prejudice against the overweight and obese. If you notice an overweight guest who's looking uncomfortable at a social event, approach him and start a conversation. Let your old way of thinking guide you to a place of compassion and kindness for others.

Sometimes people who've lost weight are unable to see themselves as "slim" or "fit." They look in a mirror and see fat where there is none, or they focus on an aspect of their body that hasn't changed with weight loss, such as a weak chin or protruding ears. This body image disturbance can be resolved with the help of a trained therapist.

> **GET PSYCHED**
>
> "A couple of years after losing my extra weight, I was putting on makeup in the mirror and suddenly burst into tears. I was so happy to have the old me back."
> —Julie, 42, Indiana

Handling Friends and Strangers

Chris S. of Oceanside, New York, notices that nearly everyone, especially strangers, treats her differently now that she's 104 pounds lighter. She recalls a recent trip to a drugstore where she asked a clerk if they had a certain product in stock. He actually walked her to the front of the store to point out the product. "Had I been 100 pounds heavier," she says, "I know the answer would have been, 'No, we don't have any' and that would have been that." In another case, she bumped into a man while bending down to pick up some yogurt at the grocery store. When she apologized, he smiled at her and said, "You can bump into me *any* time."

"I know had I been 100 pounds heavier, I would have gotten a dirty look," Chris says. "My personality hasn't changed. I didn't change my hair or eye color. I just changed my size. Now the whole world is looking at me differently. It's just unbelievable. I laugh now, it's so funny."

Chris continues, "For 36 years, I've been overweight. People are not nice to you when you're overweight and

> **WEB TALK:** For an interesting look at how your beliefs about overweight and obese can be measured, take the Implicit Association Test at:
> https://implicit.harvard.edu/implicit/demo/

schlepping your kids around. You're ignored, or they say cruel things to you. Now I'm seeing that I'm treated differently, and it's hard to change my way of thinking."

When we lose weight, we find out that what we suspected all along—that people treat others based on how they look—is indeed true. In some people, this confirmation can drum up anger. Here are some points to consider:

- Step back and look at the situation. Did the person who's treating you "differently" know you when you were over-weight, or are you assuming you're being treated differently by a stranger just because you're no longer overweight?

- If you're now fielding a lot of attention from others, could it be because you have changed your behaviors in some way? Perhaps you are more outgoing than you used to be, which makes you more approachable.

- If the attention bothers you—for example, a person who used to make fun of you behind your back now wants to be your best buddy—you can choose to ignore it. Seek out those people who enjoy your company because of who you are.

- Accept that looks are one of the ways we're initially attracted to others. Likewise, looks can also turn us off from other people. When we're open-minded, we try to go beyond those first impressions to forge deeper connections with people we may have dismissed out of hand.

Jealousy When you lose weight and feel happy with your appearance, you expect that everyone else will be happy, too. Unfortunately, many dieters learn that weight loss brings out a lot of ugly feelings in the people they are closest to. One of those feelings is jealousy.

Susan Jeffers, Ph.D., author of *Feel the Fear and Do It Anyway*, had a client who had lost a lot of weight and who was concerned because her partner felt threatened. "Now she was attractive and getting a lot of attention," says Jeffers, and that was disturbing to her partner. It caused some real difficulty in their relationship, although luckily they were able to work through it.

"If your partner [or friend] does show some discomfort over your weight loss," says Jeffers, "it isn't a sign the relationship is on the rocks. It's normal to have fears and feelings like this."

Jeffers offers these tips for dealing with jealousy:

- First, it's most important to take responsibility for your health. Staying overweight so your partner or friend won't feel threatened isn't good for your physical or mental health. Remind this person that you're losing weight and getting in shape because your health was at stake, not your relationship.

- Have compassion for the person who is feeling threatened. Jealousy is a normal emotion. Give the person reassurance that you love them or care for them and your weight loss doesn't change your feelings.

- Pledge to help each other be the best you can be.

- Prepare to walk away from people who don't want you to be the best you can be. That's a scary idea to most people, admits Jeffers. "You have to believe if anything happens to the relationship, you'll be able to handle it," she says.

Weight loss often shows you who your true friends are. You may discover that a friend who loved being with you when you were overweight no longer wants to hang out with you. When you were overweight, she may have felt it gave her an edge on male attention. She could feel better about herself when she stood next to you at the bar. Now when you go out with her, she feels she has to compete with you. She doesn't like it that guys are coming over to you to ask for a dance and ignoring her. Rather than tell you how she feels, she may start making hurtful comments about your looks or the "suggestive" clothes you can now comfortably wear. Or she may abandon your friendship outright because she no longer has any use for someone who can't play the role in her drama.

Obviously, if the latter happens, you've just found out what kind of friend you had. But if it's someone you truly care about, accept that jealousy is normal. Talk with your friend about her feelings. Remind her that you're her friend through "thick or thin."

GET PSYCHED

"It is part of prudence to be on the lookout for people and situations that could sabotage your new way of life." –*Victoria Moran in* Fit from Within

Romance Many overweight or obese people have lived with people close to them saying, "She'd be so pretty if she just lost a few pounds," or "Such a handsome guy under all that weight. What a catch he'd be if he was thinner." Now the weight is gone, and suddenly, other people notice the pretty girl or the handsome guy, including potential romantic partners.

Sudden romantic attention or even aesthetic appreciation can be rough for people who've lost weight. First, they may be confused. *Why is this person interested in me? Is this a joke? Are they just making fun of me?*

You may also not know how to behave. Some formerly overweight people dive into relationships because after years of being ashamed of their bodies, they're ready to explore what they feel has been denied them—intimacy, romance, and great sex. They can often feel like giddy teenagers again, exulting in their new-found sexual powers and skills of attraction. They can become promiscuous or involved in relationships that are not good for them. If the successful dieter is in a relationship, he or she may be tempted to cheat on their partner, to "test the waters" as it were.

Then there's the anger. If you were always the person who was ignored at a dance and now the guys who used to shun you call morning, noon, and night, you may be thinking, *You didn't like me before. I'm still the same person I was inside. Just because I'm thin, you like me now?* It brings out all the prejudices and stereotypes about overweight front and center. It can be terribly hurtful to really see how you were treated in the past when you were overweight.

If you find the attention you're getting flattering, there's no need to agonize over it. Enjoy it. Go out on dates. Reconnect with your spouse. Be flirtatious with the guy bagging your groceries.

But if you find yourself being pulled into risky situations—sex with multiple partners, for example, or you're thinking about having an affair with a woman at work who has been giving you every signal that she thinks you're hot—it's time to talk to someone. Sexual promiscuity can turn into an addiction. You may be replacing sex and intimacy for your old food addiction. And breaking a vow of trust with someone is never right. If you're thinking of cheating, it's time to take a hard look at your relationship with your partner and decide either to work on it or end it.

Sweet Rewards

Rewarding yourself during your weight-loss program probably helped you stay motivated, especially if you had a lot of weight to lose. Did you buy yourself a new wardrobe after losing 50 pounds? Perhaps when you finally got over a weight plateau you treated yourself to a massage. Or maybe for every week you ate your veggies, you rewarded yourself with a trip to the bookstore.

you're not alone

By the time I was 15, I weighed more than 171 pounds. I stopped weighing myself at that point. I was picked on in school and wasn't the happiest person on the planet. I tried every diet in the world, and nothing seemed to work because I always felt deprived or that I'd never be able to follow a diet forever. If I went off the diet *du jour*, I'd end up eating even more 'bad foods' with a vow to 'start over tomorrow' rather than just getting back on the plan.

By the time I was in my early 20s, I realized that I had a strong talent for cooking, so I figured I could make-over my favorite foods so I wouldn't feel deprived. I stopped dieting, and that's when I lost weight. I began to make more conscious choices about my food. If I wanted a piece of chocolate cake, I'd have it. I learned that I didn't have to eat three or four pieces of it to feel satisfied. I moved to Los Angeles after college, went to culinary school, and opened a catering business specializing in 'scrumptious cuisine for a healthy lifestyle.' A few years ago, I started writing recipe articles for national fitness magazines and started doing television guest spots to help others on a large scale learn how to make yummy, healthy food, so like me, they would no longer have to 'diet.' I recently signed a book deal for a cookbook that will teach home cooks how to make healthy versions of their favorite fast foods from places such as Dairy Queen and Kentucky Fried Chicken. I'm also in the process of signing a deal with the Food Network for a show in which I'll teach viewers how to make their favorite comfort foods with a fraction of the fat and calories. Plus, I'm the contributing food editor of the new *Women's Health* magazine.

Even though I'm around food all day long, I've retained a 55-pound weight loss for the past 12 years. If you had told me as a teen that that would be possible, I never would have believed you. I don't diet, I'm excited about waking up every morning, and I *never* feel deprived. It's so exciting to be able to show others how to do it as well! *–Devin Alexander, 33, Los Angeles, California, lost 55 pounds*

If goals and rewards motivated you to lose weight, there's no reason for you to give them up. Maintaining your ideal weight will also take work, so why not continue to make the process pleasurable?

For every month you maintain your weight, treat yourself to a new item of clothing that shows off your new shape: a flirty skirt or some sexy, strappy heels, if you're proud of your legs, or pants that require a belt.

Promise yourself that after a year of maintaining your weight, you'll take a trip to a destination you've always wanted to visit: Cancun, Europe, or a cruise in the Caribbean.

Do something you never imagined yourself doing when you were overweight or obese. Train for and run in a 5K road race. Take trapeze lessons. Join an online dating service.

If you're feeling confident you can continue to maintain the weight loss, try eliminating another health challenge in your life, such as smoking. Many of the skills you've learned while overcoming overeating and lack of exercise can be applied to other health challenges. Use a solid reward system to keep you motivated to change this habit.

> **WEB TALK:** If you've lost 30 pounds or more and kept it off for more than a year, become one of the success stories at the NWCR:
>
> www.nwcr.ws/NWCR_join.htm

Cosmetic Surgery

Some people, especially after a significant weight loss, find their body doesn't automatically bounce back into shape and no amount of exercise can tone the muscles and loose skin. Someone who was morbidly obese, for example, may have dozens of pounds of loose skin on his body, and the only way to remove it is through surgery. Another person may find that weight loss makes him look older; his jowls may be more pronounced, the skin on his neck sags, and his face appears more wrinkled. He may have a hot new body, but his face makes him look 20 years older than he really is.

That's when plastic surgery can help. The American Society of Plastic Surgeons reports that in 2004, 55,927 body-contouring procedures were performed on patients after massive weight loss—an increase of about 7 percent from 2003.

Sagging and drooping occurs because over time, the skin on the body is under a great deal of tension from the fat underneath the skin. When skin is young, healthy, and pliable, it bounces back into shape when the fat underneath disappears. But often that skin has been under tension so long, it loses the ability to bounce back. Sagging can occur anywhere, but it usually occurs on the parts of the body where fat tends to collect, such as the abdomen, breasts, upper arms, thighs, neck, and chin. Sagging isn't the only cosmetic problem with losing weight; some people also get stretch marks on their skin.

Skin also sags because of age. The younger you are, the more likely your skin is to bounce back. Sagging also depends on how much weight you've lost. A loss of a dozen pounds probably doesn't have much effect on sagging; your skin will bounce back easily. But a loss of hundreds of pounds, especially when the weight has come off rather quickly—such as through gastric bypass surgery—can create immense amounts of sagging. Other sag factors include heredity, skin tone, sun damage, and cigarette smoking.

WEB TALK: For an excellent overview on the types of cosmetic surgery available after weight loss, visit:

www.obesityhelp.com/morbidobesity/plastsurg.phtm

Many people don't feel their weight-loss journey is complete until all physical reminders of their overweight, such as the sagging breasts or flabby skin, are diminished. If you feel this way, then, by all means, investigate what solutions plastic surgery can offer you.

Q & A

Will my health insurance cover my tummy tuck?

It depends. According to the American Society of Plastic Surgeons, insurance companies generally cover reconstructive surgical procedures used to correct abnormal structures of the body caused by congenital defects, developmental abnormalities, trauma, infection, tumors, or disease. Coverage can vary from plan to plan. However, surgical procedures that are undertaken to improve a patient's appearance or self-esteem, typically known as plastic surgery, are usually not covered.

But there are "gray areas" that make such black-and-white determinations difficult. For example, someone who has 25 pounds of excess skin on her body after weight loss may have chronic infections in the skin folds that can only be alleviated through surgical removal of the skin. Her doctor may determine the surgery is medically necessary and, thus, the insurance company may decide to cover the cost.

In any case, when you make an appointment with a plastic surgeon, bring your insurance information with you. Your surgeon can advise you what your chances of having the procedure covered are and what options you have for payment. For more information on insurance coverage, see www.plasticsurgery.org/public_education/procedures/insurance_coverage.cfm.

As with losing weight, plastic surgery will not fix a bad marriage or cure your emotional problems, but it can certainly be a boost to your self-esteem. No amount of plastic surgery can change your life, and no procedure will ever make you look "perfect." If you're being treated for depression or another mental disorder, a good plastic surgeon will want you to wait until treatment is completed before considering surgery. Your body can develop some scarring, as well as other side effects because of the surgery. And as with any surgery, there are no guarantees you'll get through it without complications.

WEB TALK: For a list of questions to ask your plastic surgeon, check out:

www.plasticsurgery.org/find_a_plastic_surgeon/What-Questions-Should-I-Ask.cfm

For a referral to a board-certified plastic surgeon, call the American Society of Plastic Surgeons at 1-888-475-2784.

Keeping the Weight Off Forever

If you've gotten this far, you've probably gotten into a groove with your eating plan. With any luck, you enjoy the way you're eating and how you feel after you exercise. As you transition to a maintenance plan, you really don't have to change things all that much if you're close to or at your goal weight. You're at your *set point*, a metabolic rate that will work to keep you at your current weight. You can continue to eat sensibly, exercise regularly, and keep an eye on how you feel and how your clothes fit to stay within your set point.

PsychSpeak

Your **set point** is the weight range your body is programmed to weigh, the weight your body naturally wants to weigh. Your set point is controlled by genetics and biology, and the only way it can be determined is by healthful eating and regular exercise. After years of dieting, your body may take up to a year to adjust to its normal metabolism.

But you can't go back to eating the way you used to eat when you were overweight or obese. You may be able to indulge more than you did when you first started dieting, but you must remain ever vigilant. Anyone who has lost weight and kept it off never forgets that weight maintenance is a permanent condition. You don't have to live a life of deprivation, but if you want to retain your new shape, you must develop markers that tell you when you're slipping out of your range.

A good measure is to try to keep your weight within a 5-pound range. If you've reached your goal weight of 170, aim for 168 to 173. If your weight starts creeping toward 174 or 175, adjust your food intake and exercise accordingly until you get back into your range. It's a good idea to weigh yourself once a week at the same time of day in the same conditions; body weights can fluctuate by a couple pounds each day, never mind day-to-day. For example, my weekly weigh-ins occur on Monday mornings, after I've emptied my bladder and before I've hopped into the shower. This way if I'm over my range weight, I can take care of it during the week, rather than over the weekend, when I tend to enjoy my treats. But your day, time, and conditions may be different. Think about what works best for your life, schedule, and patterns.

Other people use their clothing as a maintenance gauge. They have a pair of pants or jeans that fit perfectly. When they start putting on weight, the pants or jeans start feeling a little uncomfortable. This discomfort signals that it's time to cut back on calories for a few days or weeks, or perhaps more exercise is in order.

> ## GET PSYCHED
>
> "I've found it's better to look at my weight as a long-term commitment rather than a phase or 'diet.' Maintaining is never really over. It does become second nature, and you subconsciously learn what you have to do to prevent weight gain, but it's still something that you must deal with, plan for, and think about frequently."
> —*Jennifer N., Jacksonville, Florida, maintaining a 40-pound weight loss for 2 years*

Jan, 48, has always been slim. At 5'7", she weighed 110 pounds when she married in her mid-20s. The Manchester, Connecticut, mother gained a few more pounds after two pregnancies, but noticed she could eat sensibly, exercise, indulge in the occasional treat, and still maintain a normal weight.

But in the last 2 years, Jan has gained 8 pounds. She hadn't changed her diet, but a knee injury had kept her from jogging. She took up walking as the injury healed, but reduced exercise aside, she places most of the blame on aging. "Keeping my weight down is much harder as I get older," she says.

Jan adds, "I've just become more aware that I have to watch things more closely. Before I went on vacation recently, I started adding exercise tapes to my workouts, or I'd run up and down stairs." Her knee injury has healed so she can now jog, but she has also taken up kayaking to help burn calories. So far, the adjustments are working. Maintaining at 125 pounds, Jan's well within the normal range of weight for her height.

Which brings us to the next point: you must keep moving if you want to keep the weight off. In a 2002 article published in the *American Journal of Clinical Nutrition*, researchers looked at the energy expenditures of 47 premenopausal women who were in their normal weight range. Half of the group were "post-obese" after successful weight loss, but all subjects were sedentary and exercised less than once a week.

A year later, researchers studied the women and looked at their body composition, physical fitness, energy exercise economy, and muscle strength. They found two groups of women, 20 of whom they labeled "gainers" because they'd put on an average of 9.6 kilograms or 21 pounds, and 27 who they labeled "maintainers," who'd only gained an average of .7 kilograms or 1.5 pounds. The maintainers showed a 44 percent higher energy expenditure over the gainers, suggesting that physical inactivity, rather than metabolism or diet, contributed to the weight gain. The authors concluded that for the gainers to catch up to the maintainers, they'd have to engage in 80 minutes per day of moderate physical activity— more than twice the amount suggested by the USDA to maintain weight loss.

If eating less and moving more doesn't get you back into your weight range, it may be time to take out your journal and start monitoring your food intake and exercise patterns. Are you slipping back into old emotional eating patterns such as snacking when you're stressed? Or perhaps you've gone back to an old habit such as eating meals absentmindedly in front of the television, which is causing you to eat more than you thought.

What You Can Do

You've attained something that millions of people in America want: permanent weight loss. It took a lot of hard work to achieve this goal—there were times when you would have rather snacked than sweated, or weeks when the scale wouldn't budge. Still, you kept at it. You've done something to be proud of. Better yet, you've probably discovered some amazing things about yourself and are ready to tackle some new challenges.

- ☐ Celebrate your weight loss! You've reached a goal elusive to many people. You worked hard. You deserve to be proud of your effort.

- ☐ Buy and wear clothes that flatter your new shape. Avoid reaching for the clothing styles you used to wear when you were heavier, such as caftans and baggy workout clothes.

- ☐ Thank the people who supported you on your journey: the co-workers who walked with you every day, rain or shine; your spouse, who gave up Krispy Kreme doughnuts just for you (good for him!); your children, who learned to enjoy a fresh salad with you every night (and good for them!).

- ☐ Create a scrapbook or make a memory box of your weight-loss journey. Include your weight-loss journal, photographs of your progress, and memories of how you felt at certain stages.

- ☐ Donate your old clothes to charity.

- ☐ Get a professional portrait taken of you at your new, permanent weight.

☐ You may look different to other people now—even your-self sometimes—but you're basically the same person you were before. Go gentle on yourself when you're feeling frustrated or confused.

☐ Make a list of all the things you wanted to do when you were overweight—and start doing them now!

☐ Keep up the good work. When your priority is to keep your body healthy, chances are you won't have to worry about your weight again.

Glossary

adrenal glands   Two endocrine glands located near the kidneys that produce and release several hormones, including adrenaline.

adrenaline   A hormone produced by the adrenal gland during intense emotional states. It stimulates the heart and nervous system, prepping the body for action.

aerobic   Literally means "with oxygen." Aerobic exercise produces energy with the oxygen in the bloodstream; it burns fat and strengthens the heart and lungs.

alternative therapy   A therapy that falls beyond the scope of traditional treatments. Acupuncture and meditation may be considered alternative therapies.

amino acid   The basic building block of protein.

anabolic   A metabolic condition in which new cells are synthesized or grown.

anorexia nervosa   An eating disorder marked by obsessive, restrictive eating, often to a point close to starvation, to feel a sense of control over the body.

appetite   An internal sensation of wanting or craving food.

appetite suppressant   A substance that curbs the feeling of hunger.

autonomic nervous system   The part of the nervous system that regulates involuntary body functions such as heart rate, blood pressure, and glandular function.

bariatric surgery   A surgical procedure used to remedy obesity.

bariatrics   The science and study of obesity.

basal metabolic rate   The energy the body needs to maintain itself at rest.

behavior modification   A technique for promoting the frequency of desirable behaviors and decreasing the incidence of unwanted ones.

behavioral therapy   The treatment used to help patients substitute desirable responses and behavior patterns for undesirable ones.

binge eating disorder   A condition characterized by eating large amounts of food even when not hungry and feeling as though the behavior is out of control.

blood sugar   Glucose in the bloodstream.

body fat percentage   The percentage of body weight that is composed of fat.

body mass index (BMI)   A formula used to measure body weight relative to height.

bulimia   An eating disorder characterized by binge eating, followed by vomiting or purging.

calorie   A unit of heat equal to the energy it takes to raise the temperature of 1 gram of water by 1 degree Celsius.

cardiovascular exercise (cardio)   Exercise involving the heart and circulatory system.

catabolic   A metabolic process that breaks down muscle to release energy.

central nervous system   The brain and spinal cord.

cholesterol   Cholesterol, a fatlike substance, is both made by the body and found in animal foods. Within the body, cholesterol is also known as a lipid. Increased cholesterol levels circulating in the bloodstream raise the risk of heart disease.

cognitive therapy   A form of therapy based on the theory that thoughts control behaviors and emotions.

commercial weight-loss program   A weight-loss program that's run as a business. Weight Watchers and Jenny Craig are examples of commercial weight-loss programs.

comorbidities   Medical problems that co-exist with a primary medical diagnosis. Insulin resistance would be considered a comorbidity to obesity.

cortisol   A hormone that is made in the adrenal glands in response to stress and which influences glucose metabolism.

crash diet   A diet that promotes rapid weight loss; when the diet ends, the weight is usually regained.

depression   A mental disorder marked by feelings of sadness, discouragement, and despair. Depression can be mild or veryserious. When untreated, extreme cases can lead to suicide.

detox diet   A diet that cleanses the body's internal organs.

diet   A prescribed selection of foods or the act of restricting food intake.

diuretics   Substances that cause the body to eliminate water.

eating disorder   A broad term covering a number of mental disorders related to eating, including anorexia nervosa, bulimia, and binge eating disorder. Eating disorders should be evaluated, diagnosed, and treated by a medical professional.

eating trigger   A mood, emotion, or situation that drives eating.

emotional eating   Characterized by excessive eating in the presence of anger, boredom, sadness, or even happiness.

empty calories   Foods that have little or no nutritional value. Soda and candy are examples of foods full of empty calories.

endorphins   Neurotransmitters that alleviate pain and provide a sense of well-being; also called "nature's opiates."

enzymes   Proteins that assist with chemical reactions in the body.

essential fatty acids (EFAs)   EFAs are nutrients that assist with everything from basic metabolic functions to possibly preventing chronic disease. They are required in the human diet because they can't be synthesized by the body—they must be obtained from food. Omega-3s and omega-6s are EFAs that can be found in vegetable oils, nuts, fish, seeds, and some leafy vegetables.

fad diet   A diet that has little or no scientific data backing it. Fad diets are usually short-term and don't produce lasting weight loss.

fasting   The act of giving up food for a period of time, usually for a day but sometimes for longer.

fats   One of the three main nutrients in food. Fats are essential for protecting organs, absorbing fat-soluble vitamins, regulating hormones, and providing energy.

fiber   A substance in plant foods that helps in the digestive process. It can also lower cholesterol and help control blood sugar.

food combining   A diet that advises eating certain types of foods at specific times.

free radical   An atom or molecule that has been rendered unstable or highly reactive because of its unpaired electron. The atom or molecule grabs electrons from molecules in healthy cells, thus damaging the cell. Free radicals are linked to aging, heart disease, and cancer.

gene   A unit of hereditary information that contains the functional and physical characteristics passed from parent to offspring. It is contained on a chromosome within the cell's nucleus.

glucose   A simple sugar made by the body from carbohydrates. It's the body's primary source of fuel.

glycemic index   A measure of a food's ability to raise blood sugar levels. Foods low on the index raise blood sugars minimally, whereas foods high on the index raise blood sugars greatly. A steady diet of high-glycemic foods can promote obesity and diabetes.

glycogen   A stored form of glucose found in the liver and muscles. The body breaks down glycogen into lactic acid.

hormone   A chemical substance formed in one part of the body that is carried by the bloodstream to affect change in another part of the body.

hunger   A physiological need for food.

hypertension   High blood pressure.

hypothalamus   The part of the brain that controls appetite.

ideal body weight/ideal size   A weight that is appropriate and healthful based on height.

inertia   The tendency of matter to remain at rest.

insulin   A hormone produced in the pancreas that helps the body metabolize glucose.

ketosis   A state of having abnormally high levels of ketones in the bloodstream, produced when the body metabolizes fat for energy. Ketosis is a common side effect of low-carbohydrate diets.

lipids   Fatty substances found in the bloodstream and body tissues. Cholesterol and triglycerides are lipids.

liposuction   A cosmetic surgery procedure in which fat is removed from the body by means of suction.

liquid diet   An extremely low-calorie diet in liquid form. Usually these diets are supervised by a health professional.

macronutrients   Nutrients the body needs in large amounts, including protein, carbohydrates, water, fats, and calcium.

metabolic syndrome   A group of metabolic risk factors that put a person at risk for coronary heart disease, stroke, type 2 diabetes, and other health conditions. Risk factors include obesity, high triglyceride levels, low HDL cholesterol levels, and high blood pressure, among others.

metabolism   The physical and chemical processes the body uses to create energy.

micronutrients   Nutrients needed in trace amounts to sustain good health, such as iron and selenium.

minerals   Inorganic substances having a definite chemical structure. The body requires minerals in small amounts through diet or supplementation.

morbid obesity   A clinical term indicating a BMI greater than 40.

net carbs   A food's total carbohydrates minus fiber, glycerin, and sugar alcohols. It is a marketing phrase used to highlight a lower carb count, not a government or scientific term.

neurotransmitter   A chemical released as a nerve impulse transmits information from one nerve cell to another.

nutrients   Elements and compounds necessary for life, including proteins, carbohydrates, fats, vitamins, and minerals.

obesity   A clinical term indicating a BMI greater than 30.

opiates   A class of drugs that depresses the central nervous system and relieves pain.

opioids   Naturally occurring chemicals in the brain that may reduce pain and induce sleep.

OTC   Acronym for "over-the-counter." OTC drugs do not require a prescription from a physician.

overweight   A clinical term indicating a BMI between 25 and 29.9.

pedometer   A mechanical device that measures the number of footsteps taken.

peer support   Support given by people who have a shared history or background. They are usually not professionals.

phytonutrients   Naturally occurring compounds found in fruits and vegetables. Phytonutrients are responsible for enhancing immunity and strengthening the heart and blood vessels.

plastic surgery   Elective surgery used to improve appearance. Many formerly obese people undergo plastic surgery to remove excess skin after weight loss.

plateau   A normal stage in the dieting process in which the body stops losing weight. Plateaus are usually temporary.

protein   A molecule composed of amino acids. The body's cells need protein to grow and mend themselves.

psychotherapist   A therapist who deals with mental and emotional disorders.

recommended dietary allowance (RDA)   A guideline to dietary intake recommended by the federal government for essential nutrients.

registered dietician (RD)   A food and nutrition expert who has met set criteria by the American Dietetic Association to earn the credential "R.D."

resistance training   Exercise that forces muscles to work against a weight. Lifting dumbbells is an example of resistance training.

"runner's high"   A common experience occurring among regular exercisers when the body releases endorphins in response to intense activity; the exerciser reports feeling joyful and happy, often for hours afterward.

satiety   The feeling of being full and satisfied after eating.

saturated fat   A type of dietary fat found in animal products that raises cholesterol levels. Saturated fats tend to be solid at room temperature. A healthy diet limits the amount of saturated fats.

sedentary   Not physically active. Someone who is sedentary is at risk for many health conditions.

serotonin   A neurotransmitter found in the brain affecting many functions, including mood, sleep, and aggression. Low levels of serotonin are associated with depression.

starvation   The act of depriving of food over a period of time.

strength training   Exercise that helps build muscle strength.

stretching   A form of exercise that stretches and elongates the muscles, promoting flexibility and injury prevention.

syndrome X   A combination of health conditions that puts a person at risk for heart disease. Conditions include type 2 diabetes, high blood pressure, and obesity. More often called "metabolic syndrome."

synthesize   To make a chemical from constituent parts.

target heart rate   The ideal number of heartbeats per minute for aerobic exercise. This number is determined by age and fitness level.

testimonial   A statement of benefits received. Testimonials are often used in the advertising of weight-loss products and programs to influence consumers.

thermogenic   Literally, "producing heat." Usually used in ad copy describing "fat-burning" OTC (over-the-counter) weight-loss supplements.

trans fatty acid (trans fat)   A fat made by transforming a liquid fat into solid fat through a chemical process called hydrogenation. Eating a diet high in trans fats raises blood cholesterol levels and increases the risk for heart disease.

triglyceride   A fatty substance in the blood that is a stored form of energy. Elevated triglyceride levels may be caused by food or alcohol and can signal a risk for heart disease.

unsaturated fats   Also called "good fats," these fats come from vegetable sources and are liquid in form at room temperature. They can lower cholesterol levels and promote heart health.

vegan   A person who does not eat or use any animal products, including meat, eggs, dairy, or fish.

vegetarian diet   A plant-based diet.

vitamins   Organic molecules obtained from foods that are necessary for normal growth, development, and maintenance of the body.

waist-to-hip ratio   The ratio of a person's waist circumference to hip circumference, indicative of risk for heart disease.

water weight loss   When the body sheds water over fat; diets that are too restrictive tend to cause the body to lose water. This is because the body holds on to fat stores when it feels it is being starved.

weight-bearing exercise   Any exercise that makes muscles or bones work against gravity, such as walking or stair climbing. Weight-bearing exercise can help prevent the loss of bone density, as well as contribute to weight loss.

weight-loss program   A system or plan designed to help lose a set amount of weight.

yo-yo dieting   A pattern of losing and gaining weight on a variety of diets. Yo-yo dieters usually can't maintain weight loss.

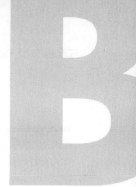

Further Reading

Many of the expert sources interviewed for this book have written their own books on subjects ranging from weight loss and exercise to overcoming habits and changing behaviors. Literally hundreds of books on weight loss, exercise, and the psychology of eating are on bookstore shelves. This reading list is by no means comprehensive.

Abramson, Edward. *Body Intelligence*. New York: McGraw-Hill, 2005.

———. *Emotional Eating: What You Need to Know Before Starting Your Next Diet*. San Francisco: Jossey-Bass, 1998.

———. *Marriage Made Me Fat!: Understand Your Weight Gain—And Lose Pounds Permanently*. New York: Kensington, 2000.

American Heart Association. *Fitting in Fitness: Hundreds of Simple Ways to Put More Physical Activity into Your Life*. New York: Clarkson Potter, 1997.

Bingham, John. *The Courage to Start: A Guide to Running for Your Life*. New York: Fireside, 1999.

Brownell, Kelly. *Food Fight: The Inside Story of the Food Industry, America's Obesity Crisis, and What We Can Do About It*. New York: McGraw-Hill, 2003.

Campbell, T. Colin, and Thomas Campbell. *The China Study: Startling Implications for Diet, Weight Loss and Long-term Health*. Dallas: BenBella, 2005.

Dorfman, Lisa. *The Vegetarian Sports Nutrition Guide: Peak Performance for Everyone from Beginners to Gold Medalists*. Hoboken, New Jersey: Wiley, 1999.

Flancbaum, Louis, Erica Manfred, and Deborah Flancbaum. *The Doctor's Guide to Weight Loss Surgery: How to Make the Decision That Could Save Your Life*. New York: Bantam, 2003.

Fletcher, Anne. *Thin for Life: 10 Keys to Success from People Who Have Lost Weight and Kept It Off*. New York: Houghton Mifflin, 2003.

Hark, Lisa, and Darwin Deen. *Nutrition for Life: The No-Fad, No-Nonsense Approach to Eating Well and Reaching Your Healthy Weight*. New York: DK-Adult, 2005.

Harvard Health Letter (newsletter). Published 12 times a year by Harvard Health Publications. Subscribe at www.health.harvard.edu/hhp/publication/view.do?name=L or by calling 1-877-649-9457.

Jeffers, Susan. *Feel the Fear and Do It Anyway*. New York: Ballantine Books, 1988.

Kushner, Robert F., and Nancy Kushner. *Dr. Kushner's Personality Type Diet*. New York: St. Martin's Griffin, 2004.

McQuillan, Susan. *Breaking the Bonds of Food Addiction*. Indianapolis: Alpha Books, 2004.

Moore, Thomas, Laura Svetkey, Pao-Hwa Lin, Nieri Karania, and Mark Jenkins. *The DASH Diet for Hypertension: Lower Your Blood Pressure in 14 Days—Without Drugs*. New York: Pocket, 2003.

Moran, Victoria. *Fit from Within: 101 Simple Secrets to Change Your Body and Your Life—Starting Today and Lasting Forever*. New York: Contemporary Books, 2002.

Netzer, Corinne. *The Complete Book of Food Counts*. New York: Dell, 2003.

Nonas, Cathy. *Outwit Your Weight: Fat-Proof Your Life with More Than 200 Tips, Tools, and Techniques to Help You Defeat Your Diet Danger Zones*. Emmaus, Pennsylvania: Rodale, 2002.

Peck, Paula. *Exodus from Obesity: The Guide to Long-term Success After Weight Loss Surgery*. Woodbridge, Virginia: BP Publishing, 2003.

Prochaska, James, John Norcross, and Carlo DiClemente. *Changing for Good. A Revolutionary Six-Stage Program for Overcoming Bad Habits and Moving Your Life Positively Forward.* New York: Perennial Currents, 1995.

Schiller, Eric, and the American Diabetes Association. *The Official Pocket Guide to Diabetic Exchanges.* Alexandria, Virginia: American Diabetes Association, 2003.

Schlosser, Eric. *Fast Food Nation: The Dark Side of the All-American Meal.* New York: Perennial, 2002.

Shell, Ellen Ruppel. *The Hungry Gene: The Science of Fat and the Future of Thin.* New York: Atlantic Monthly Press, 2002.

Tufts University Health & Nutrition Letter. Published 12 times a year by Tufts Media. Subscribe at healthletter.tufts.edu/ or by calling 1-800-274-7581.

University of California, Berkeley Wellness Letter. Published 12 times a year by Health Letter Associates. Subscribe at www.wellnessletter.com/ or by calling 1-800-829-9170.

Willett, Walter. *Eat, Drink, and Be Healthy: The Harvard Medical School Guide to Healthy Eating.* New York: Free Press, 2002.

Williams, Jayne. *Slow Fat Triathlete: Live Your Athletic Dreams in the Body You Have Now.* New York: Marlowe and Company, 2004.

Resources

n addition to the many books you can read about weight loss, exercise, and health, there are literally dozens of organizations, websites, and weight-loss support options that can provide additional support and help. Here is just a sampling of them.

Weight-Loss Information

Aim for a Healthy Weight
www.nhlbi.nih.gov/health/public/
heart/obesity/lose_wt/index.htm

American Cancer Society
1599 Clifton Road NE
Atlanta, GA 30329
1-800-ACS-2345 (1-800-227-2345)
www.cancer.org

American Diabetes Association
ATTN: National Call Center
1701 North Beauregard Street
Alexandria, VA 22311
1-800-DIABETES (1-800-342-2383)
www.diabetes.org or www.diabetes.
org/weightloss-and-exercise.jsp

American Dietetic Association
120 South Riverside Plaza, Suite
2000
Chicago, IL 60606-6995
1-800-877-1600
www.eatright.org

American Heart Association
National Center
7272 Greenville Avenue
Dallas, TX 75231
1-800-AHA-USA-1 (1-800-242-8721)
www.americanheart.org/

American Obesity Association
1250 24th Street, NW, Suite 300
Washington, DC 20037
www.obesity.org

**American Society for Bariatric
Surgery**
100 SW 75th Street, Suite 201
Gainesville, FL 32607
www.asbs.org/

**American Society of Bariatric
Physicians**
2821 S. Parker Road, Suite 625
Aurora, CO 80014
www.asbp.org/

FDA's Overweight and Obesity Website
www.fda.gov/oc/opacom/
hottopics/obesity.html

Healthier US.gov
healthierus.gov/

Joslin Diabetes Center
One Joslin Place
Boston, MA 02215
617-732-2400
www.joslin.org

MedLinePlus: Obesity
www.nlm.nih.gov/medlineplus/
obesity.html
(Provides links to dozens of government-related weight-loss resources.)

**National Heart, Lung, and Blood Institute
Obesity Education Initiative**
PO Box 30105
Bethesda, MD 20824-0105
www.nhlbi.nih.gov/about/oei/
index.htm

National Weight Control Registry
www.nwcr.ws/

Physicians Committee for Responsible Medicine
5100 Wisconsin Avenue, N.W., Suite 400
Washington, DC 20016
202-686-2210
www.pcrm.org/health/prevmed/
weight_control.html

Weight Control and Obesity Topic Page
www.nal.usda.gov/fnic/etext/
000060.html
(Part of the USDA's Food and Nutrition Information Center)

Weight-Control Information Network (WIN)
1 WIN Way
Bethesda, MD 20892
877-946-4627
win.niddk.nih.gov/

World Health Organization
Regional Office for the Americas
525 23rd Street, N.W.
Washington, DC 20037
202-974-3000
www.who.int or www.who.int/
topics/obesity/en/

Specific Diets

Atkins Nutritionals
2002 Orville Dr. North, Suite A
Ronkonkoma, NY 11779-7661
1-800-2-ATKINS (1-800-228-5467)
atkins.com

Calorie Restriction (CR) Society
1827 W. 145th Street, Suite 205
Gardena, CA 90249
1-800-929-6511
www.calorierestriction.org

Dean Ornish, M.D.'s Lifestyle Program
my.webmd.com/content/pages/9/
3068_9408.htm

Diet.com
Diet Health, Inc.
50 First Street, Suite 603
San Francisco, CA 94105
www.diet.com
(Dr. Robert Kushner's personality-type diet)

eDiets.com
3801 W. Hillsboro Blvd.
Deerfield Beach, FL 33442
954-360-9022
www.ediets.com

Jenny Craig International
5770 Fleet Street
Carlsbad, CA 92008
1-800-597-JENNY (1-800-597-5366)
www.jennycraig.com

LA Weight Loss
1-800-331-4035
www.laweightloss.com

NutriSystem
200 Welsh Road
Horsham, PA 19044
1-800-321-THIN (1-800-321-8446)
www.nutrisystem.com

The Paleolithic Diet Page
www.paleodiet.com/

Pritikin
The Yacht Club at Turnberry Isle
19735 Turnberry Way
Aventura, FL 33180
305-935-7131 or 1-800-327-4914
www.pritikin.com

Slim-Fast
Slim-Fast Foods Company
PO Box 3625
West Palm Beach, FL 33402
561-833-9920
www.slimfast.com

South Beach Diet
www.southbeachdiet.com

Sugar Busters!
www.sugarbusters.com

The Vegetarian Resource Group
PO Box 1463
Baltimore, MD 21203
410-366-8343
www.vrg.org

The Vegetarian Society
The Vegetarian Society of the
United Kingdom
Parkdale, Dunham Road
Altrincham, Cheshire, England
WA14 4QG
0161 925 2000
www.vegsoc.org

Weight Watchers International
Weight Watchers International, Inc.
175 Crossways Park West
Woodbury, NY 11797
1-800-651-6000
www.weightwatchers.com

The Zone Diet
www.drsears.com

Hospital- and University-Based Weight-Loss Programs

The Colorado Weigh Program
University of Colorado Center
for Human Nutrition
7476 East 29th Avenue
Town Center, PMB 113
Denver, CO 80238
303-892-0128
www.coloradoweigh.com/

Duke Diet and Fitness Center
804 West Trinity Avenue
Durham, NC 27701
1-800-235-3853
www.cfl.duke.edu/
(03gujp45hlzgk345ex2rxvnk)/dfc/
home/

**The Lifespan Weight
Management Program**
167 Point Street
Providence, RI 02903
401-444-4800
www.lifespan.org/SvcLines/
BehavHealth/BehavMed/
WtMgmt.htm

**Northwestern Memorial
Hospital Wellness Institute**
150 East Huron Street, Suite 100
Chicago, IL 60611
312-926-9355
www.nmh.org/nmh/
specialtiesandservices/
servicescenters/wi/main.htm

**Pennington Biomedical
Research Center**
Division of Clinical Obesity and
Metabolic Syndrome
6400 Perkins Road
Baton Rouge, LA 70808
225-763-2500
www.pbrc.edu/
prog_obesityclinical.htm

**UCLA Risk Factor Obesity
Program**
UCLA Center for Human
Nutrition
900 Veteran Avenue
Los Angeles, CA 90095
310-825-8173
rfoweightloss.med.ucla.edu/

**University of Alabama at
Birmingham EatRight Weight
Management Program**
Kirklin Clinic
2000 6th Avenue South
Birmingham, AL 35249
205-934-7053
www.health.uab.edu/
show.asp?durki=61929

**University of Illinois Medical
Center Weight Management
Program**
1740 West Taylor Street
Chicago, IL 60612
866-600-CARE
uillinoismedcenter.org/content.
cfm/weight_loss

University of Pennsylvania
Health System's Department
of Psychiatry Weight and
Eating Disorders Program
3535 Market Street, Suite 3108
Philadelphia, PA 19104
215-898-7314
www.uphs.upenn.edu/weight/

The Weight Control Program at
the University of Vermont
Burlington, VT 05405
802-656-2661
www.uvm.edu/~psych/research/
weight_control_flyer.pdf

Yale Center for Eating and
Weight Disorders
PO Box 208205
New Haven, CT 06520
203-432-4610
www.yale.edu/ycewd/index.html

Exercise and Fitness Information

Active.com
10182 Telesis Court, Suite 300
San Diego, CA 92121
1-888-543-7223
www.active.com

American Council on Exercise
4851 Paramount Drive
San Diego, CA 92123
858-279-8227 or 1-800-825-3636
www.acefitness.org

Hearts N' Parks
PO Box 30105
Bethesda, MD 20824-0105
301-592-8573
www.nhlbi.nih.gov/health/prof/
heart/obesity/hrt_n_pk/index.htm

President's Council on Physical
Fitness and Sports
Department W
200 Independence Avenue, SW
Room 738-H
Washington, DC 20201-0004
202-690-9000
www.fitness.gov

Recreation.gov
Recreation One-Stop Initiative
Department of the Interior
Mail Stop 5258 MIB
1849 C Street NW
Washington, DC 20240
www.recreation.gov

Weight-Loss/Overweight/Obesity Support Groups

ObesityHelp.com
Association for Morbid Obesity
Support
8001 Irvine Center Drive, Suite
1270
Irvine, CA 92618-3001
866-WLS-INFO (866-957-4636)
www.obesityhelp.com

Overeaters Anonymous
World Service Office
PO Box 44020
Rio Rancho, NM 87174-4020
505-891-2664
www.oa.org

**Taking Off Pounds Sensibly
(TOPS)**
TOPS Club, Inc.
4575 South Fifth Street
PO Box 070360
Milwaukee, WI 53207-0360
414-482-4620
www.tops.org

**Trevose Behavior Modification
Program**
PO Box 11674
Philadelphia, PA 19116
www.tbmp.org/

Other Organizations

**American Psychological
Association**
APA Help Center/Eating
Disorders
750 First Street, NE
Washington, DC 20002-4242
1-800-374-2721
www.apahelpcenter.org/articles/
article.php?id=9

Eating Disorders Association
Eating Disorders Association
103 Prince of Wales Road
Norwich NR1 1DW
United Kingdom
www.edauk.com/

**National Eating Disorders
Association**
603 Stewart Street, Suite 803
Seattle, WA 98101
206-382-3587
www.nationaleatingdisorders.org

Index

A

Abramson, Edward, Ph.D., 232
accountability
  commercial restriction diets, 55
  exercise plans, 191-192
achievable goals, 160
action (stage of change), 38
acupuncture, 212
ADA (American Dietetic
  Association), 90-91
Adipex-P (phentermine), 134
adjustable gastric banding (AGB),
  138-139
aerobic exercise, 175
affirmations, 213-214
Agatston, Arthur (South Beach
  diet), 64
AGB (adjustable gastric banding),
  138-139
Agency for Healthcare Research
  and Quality, 2004 report on
  bariatric surgery, 137
aging, 13-14, 244-246
all-or-nothing thinking, 15-16
Alley, Kirstie, 116
Alt, Carol, 116
alternative therapies, 212-214
American Academy of Family
  Physicians, 315
American Academy of Pediatrics,
  315

American Dietetic Association
  (ADA), 90-91, 315
American Heart Association, 177,
  270
American Obesity Association,
  14, 313
American Society for Bariatric
  Surgery (ASBS), 135
American Society of Plastic
  Surgeons, 330, 332
angioplasty, 267
anorexia nervosa, 250
Anoxine-AM, 134
anti-cancer diet. *See* macrobiotic
  diet
antidepressants
  effects on weight, 248
  off-label use, 134
arthritis, osteoarthritis, 276-277
ASBS (American Society for
  Bariatric Surgery), 135
Asian-style diets, 93, 96
astrological sign diet, 115
at-home activities, support for
  children and teens, 313-314
atherosclerosis, 266-268
athletic diets, 89-91
Atkins diet, 61-64
Atkins, Dr. Robert, 61
attitude, 30
  adjustment traits, 43
  role of mind in weight-loss, 3-5

D

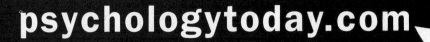